the vegan cookbook

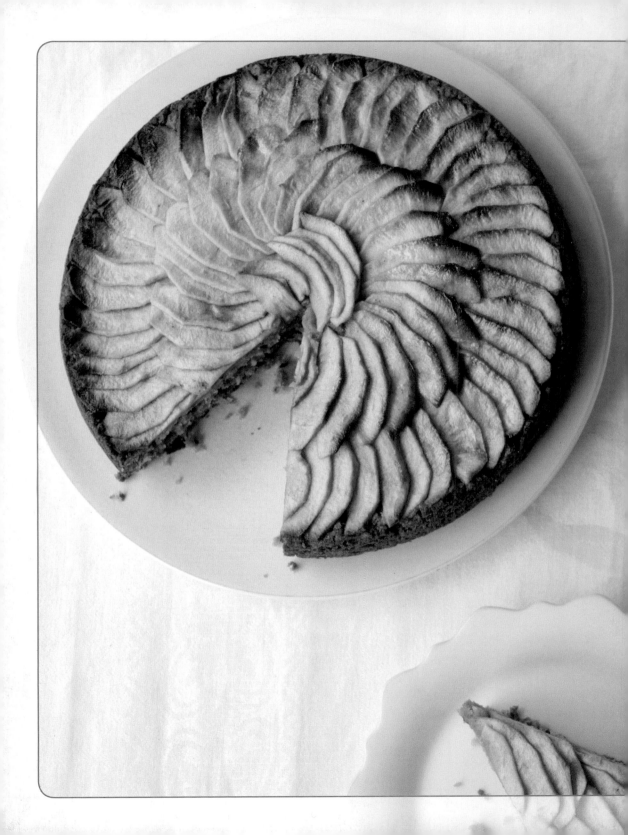

DUNCAN BAIRD PUBLISHERS
LONDON

the
vegan
cookbook

Feed Your Soul, Taste the Love:
100 of the Best Vegan Recipes

Adele McConnell

To my dear husband, Paul.

The Vegan Cookbook
Adele McConnell

First published in the USA and Canada in 2014 by
Duncan Baird Publishers, an imprint of
Watkins Publishing Limited
PO Box 883, Oxford OX1 9PL, UK

A member of Osprey Group
Osprey Publishing
PO Box 3985
New York, NY 10185-3985
Tel: (001) 212 753 4402
Email: info@ospreypublishing.com

Publisher: Grace Cheetham
Editor: Jan Cutler
Art Direction and Design: Manisha Patel
Americanizer: Delora Jones
Production: Uzma Taj
Commissioned photography: Keiko Oikawa
Food Stylist: Aya Nishimura
Prop Stylist: Lucy Harvey

ISBN: 978-1-84899-119-4

10 9 8 7 6 5 4 3 2 1

Typeset in Nobel, Beton and Biscotti
Color reproduction by PDQ, UK
Printed in China

PUBLISHER'S NOTE While every care has been taken in
compiling the recipes for this book, Watkins Publishing
Limited, or any other persons who have been involved in
working on this publication, cannot accept responsibility
for any errors or omissions, inadvertent or not, that may be
found in the recipes or text, nor for any problems that may
arise as a result of preparing one of these recipes. If you
are pregnant or breastfeeding or have any special dietary
requirements or medical conditions, it is advisable to
consult a medical professional before following any of
the recipes contained in this book.

NOTES ON THE RECIPES Unless otherwise stated:
• Use filtered water
• Use organic ingredients where possible
• Use homemade vegetable stock in preference, or use
vegan, gluten-free, dairy-free stock or cubes or granules
• Use medium fruit and vegetables, unless otherwise stated
• Use fresh ingredients, including herbs and chilies
• 1 teaspoon = 5ml. 1 tablespoon = 15ml. 1 cup = 240ml.

The food symbols refer to the recipes only, not including
ingredient alternatives, optional ingredients or serving
suggestions. Pine nuts and coconut have been classed
as nuts. Coconut sugar has been treated as a nut-free
ingredient, as it is derived from the sap rather than the
nut of the coconut palm.

Check the manufacturer's labeling, because the
ingredients used in different brands vary, especially
for small quantities of ingredients such as soy and
sugar, although manufacturers are not required to
detail minuscule quantities of ingredients.

The "Raw" symbol has been used to identify recipes made
from raw ingredients that are not heated above 98.6°F.
These recipes may sometimes contain natural sweeteners
such as agave or coconut sugar. If following a strict raw-
foods diet, look for recipes containing both the "Sugar-free"
and "Raw" symbols.

Watkins Publishing is supporting the Woodland Trust, the
UK's leading woodland conservation charity, by funding
tree-planting initiatives and woodland maintenance.

www.dbp.co.uk

Contents

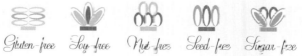

Gluten-free   Soy-free   Nut-free   Seed-free   Sugar-free   Raw

Introduction

Writing this book has been the most exciting project I've ever taken on, and it is the result of years of experimentation based on my passion for good, healthy food. I have been blogging on my website, Vegie Head, since 2010, and my recipes have been enjoyed and recreated by tens of thousands of people all over the world, in their homes, in restaurants and in cafés.

There is nothing more satisfying to me than the varied aromas of the food I love: a Mediterranean soup simmering on the stove on a cold day; the fresh smell of homebaked banana bread, still warm from the oven; curry spices being dry-fried, releasing their fragrance, and toasted sesame oil sizzling in a wok.

I was a vegetarian at 17, and I didn't eat eggs or dairy, so after ten years it was an easy step to give up the final few animal foods and become vegan. When I first moved away from home, I wanted to ensure that I was eating and enjoying a wide range of food, so I'd spend my time blending healthy smoothies and making a mess in my yellow 1960's kitchen in Melbourne. I wrote new recipes, amended old recipes to make them vegan, and changed vegan recipes to make them healthier by using coconut oil instead of margarine, homemade almond milk instead of soy milk, and by making green smoothies instead of chocolate "milkshakes."

The raw-food movement happened slowly in Australia, but I was hooked immediately. I discovered a whole new way of cooking—or not cooking—and have been excited by the challenge of trying the same foods made in a different way or clever remakes of classics that were enhanced by the health benefits of eating foods raw. Some of my first experiments were with raw cacao powder that I had bought in bulk because I had heard of its health benefits. As a chocolate lover, I have particularly enjoyed trying out new desserts, snacks and smoothies using it.

I don't want to miss out on exciting flavors just because I don't eat animal products, so I focus on delicious food from different cultures.

Whether it's Indian, Moroccan, Thai, Japanese, Vietnamese or Mexican, I've done them all, and I love them all. I adore the earthy spices and the layers of heat in Indian food, and the surprising bursts of sweetness when you bite into a dried fig or a date in Moroccan cuisine. I enjoy the creamy coconut, tangy lemongrass and that zing from kaffir lime that create the signature flavors of Thai dishes. The contrasting textures of Japanese food with its crisp tempura-batter fried vegetables, and the combination of mint and sesame in Vietnamese dishes are all part of my food experience. And then there's the food of Mexico—my beloved. Not the oily, cheese-laden Tex-Mex that's so often passed off as Mexican cooking, but real Mexican food—light, flavorsome and designed to share.

In this book I offer you a fresher, healthier approach to plant-based food—one where you will never have to lose out on flavor and variety. Whatever reason it appeals to you—your concern for animals, consideration for the Earth, or your health—you will find that a plant-based diet is easy and tastes good. You won't be told what you can't eat, but you will probably be introduced to new foods. As you adopt a new diet, you can be an example to those around you. You can change people's perspective on veganism and vegetarianism without scaring them away with statistics, facts or disturbing images, or by listing what they can't do or eat. Instead, you can show them what they can eat and that eating vegan food is an adventure in taste and ingredients.

I mentor hundreds of people all over the world on how to eat a plant-based diet—from athletes and celebrities to your neighbor down the road. They all ask me what they can eat and they are always surprised by the variety. There is no feeling of deprivation. There is only an abundance of healthy filling, incredible food.

My way of showing love to those around me is to cook. To be able to bring people together around a table and look into their faces as they savor a mouthful of food made for them is the ultimate act of giving.

For now, feed your soul and taste the love.

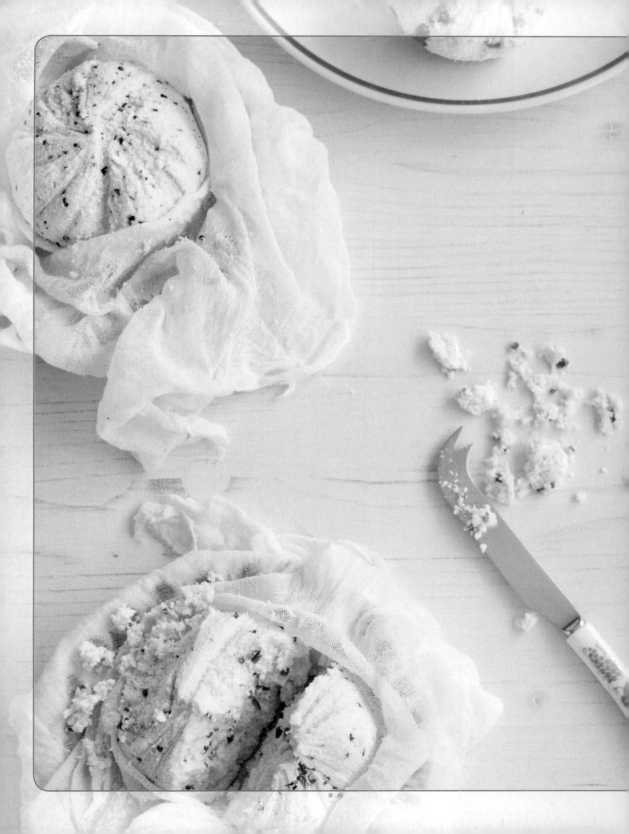

The Plant - Based Diet

A diet based on plant foods is not one of restriction or denial. You will find that there is a wide range of healthy and incredibly tasty foods that will make you feel nourished and satisfied after your meals. In the following chapter I explain the benefits of a plant-based diet and how to incorporate plant foods into your daily life. With any change of diet there will be some planning, but when you start on the recipes in this book you can use the more commonly available ingredients. You can then begin to build up a range of healthier alternatives as you become more inspired by this new way of eating.

Variations of Herbed Almond Cheese (page 22) – clockwise from top left: black pepper, apricot, chive, chili.

The Benefits of Plant Foods

Each one of us is different, and for many people a diet based on plant foods is more suitable than one that is centered on animal produce. It addresses the moral and philosophical objections that many have to eating food from animals, and there are a number of health benefits when you eat only foods made from plants.

THE PLEASURES OF A PLANT-BASED DIET

At the time of writing this book, I have followed a plant-based diet for four years and have never felt better. I sleep well, my digestion is in perfect working order, my skin is clear and my eyes are bright. My hair and nails grow super-fast and I always have tons of energy. Many people, through my blog and mentoring sessions, tell me that they have also enjoyed improved health after they have given up meat and animal produce. They are often surprised that a vegan diet can offer such a vast selection of foods and tastes, and they never miss eating meat. They have soon become completely comfortable with, and accustomed to, the fresh flavors of vegetables combined with the more sustaining vegetarian protein foods of legumes and nuts combined with grains.

As you change your diet, you will probably find that the amount of fiber you eat will increase, particularly if you had been following the standard diet of processed foods. Fiber is important for regular bowel movements and managing cholesterol levels. It also stops you from overeating. Processed foods, which are low in fiber, leave you feeling unsatisfied and prone to eating more.

Plants, nuts and seeds are high in vitamins and minerals, and when you eat a variety of them you will increase your body's opportunities to benefit from nutrients and antioxidants that it may never have had in the past. A plant-based diet is low in the type of saturated fat that might be harmful to health, but it does include coconut oil, a saturated fat known as medium chain that your body recognizes as an energy source and uses accordingly. Coconut oil is not easily stored by the body as fat.

Numerous studies have shown that people who eat a plant-based diet have lower rates of heart disease and benefit from lower blood cholesterol levels, lower blood pressure, a lower incidence of type-2 diabetes and lower rates of prostate and colon cancer, according to the American Dietetic Association.

Health benefits aside, a plant-based diet can widen your horizons for discovering a wealth of new flavors, textures, colors, tastes and culinary experiences.

RAW INGREDIENTS FOR A HEALTH BOOST

Eating some foods raw and unprocessed—in smoothies, salads, and even dessert cakes—is a great way to experiment with new, nutrient-packed ingredients. By including raw foods in your diet you will benefit from those minerals and nutrients that are lost when food is cooked or heated above 98.6°F. There are a number of raw recipes in the book. Look for the "Raw" symbol.

A RELEASE FROM SOME OF THE STRESSES IN LIFE

For me, one of the benefits of not eating animal foods is that I won't be a part of the stress that animals go through at the end of their lives—and all too frequently while being reared as well. When you eat meat, chicken or fish, you are eating those creatures' fear. You are consuming their stress, their hormones and, metaphysically, their energy.

I have realized that in order for me to live as stress-free a life as possible, I need to appreciate the intimate relationship that food has with the body, mind and spirit. Clearing my body of animal produce has allowed me to tap into a deeper level of consciousness and to have more compassion for other living beings.

CHOOSING A MEAT-FREE LIFESTYLE

One way to decide which kind of diet you might like to follow is to ask yourself, "Is this food serving me? Is this food helping me to reach my full, healthy potential? Is what I'm about to eat good for me and for the world?" You may then decide that following a vegan, or at least a meat-free, lifestyle is the right choice for you.

Plant-Based Foods for Every Day of Your Life

I explain to my clients that there are no good or bad foods when you follow a plant-based diet, but it's more about adding new ingredients to your selection and discovering the benefits of eating more raw produce. As your choices widen, so will the nutritional value of your daily diet. When you increase the good things, the less-beneficial foods take a back seat.

THE FIRST STEPS

Rather than banning foods, start to introduce new ones—for example, add almond milk to your cereal every day, and handfuls of kale or spinach to your stir-fries, pastas and soups. With just those few changes you will have increased the amount of fiber, vitamins, minerals and nutrients in your diet without really changing anything else.

If you have always drunk dairy milk, you might find nut milks a little unusual to start with, but you'll soon get to like the fresh non-dairy taste. You can make nut milks yourself, and I include a recipe in this book. Try different types of nut until you find a flavor you like.

If you can, shop at your local health-food store, organic or local produce market, or farmers' market—or even at the fresh aisles in the supermarket, keeping away from the convenience foods. Stock up on foods such as brown rice. It is satisfying, wholesome and makes a great base for meals such as curries and stews. Lentils and cannellini beans—and a wide range of other legumes—are delicious added to soups and casseroles and are an inexpensive way to bulk meals and add protein.

I choose not to use a lot of soy in my diet, but I have included some tofu and tempeh recipes in this book due to popular demand. Soy contains phytoestrogens—plant hormones that mimic estrogen in the body. Some experts claim that too much soy can be detrimental to health, so I suggest that if you choose to eat it, have it in moderation and preferably use fermented soy (miso, tempeh and tamari), which is easier to digest. I also prefer to use coconut sugar or coconut nectar rather than cane sugar. They have a lower glycemic index (GI) and do not cause a rapid increase in blood sugar levels (sugar spikes), which encourage weight gain and lead to unhealthy conditions in the body, such as diabetes.

CHOOSE PROTEIN AND NUTRIENT-RICH FOODS

Animal proteins are called complete proteins because they contain all the essential amino acids that the body cannot produce itself. Soy foods are also complete proteins. Plant foods have different amino-acid profiles, so vegans need to eat a variety of grains, legumes, nuts and seeds to meet the body's needs. These don't all have to be included in the same meal but can be eaten over the course of a day.

Eat flaxseeds and chia seeds to obtain your omega-3 essential fats. It's also important to ensure that you have enough vitamin B12, which is not available from plant foods. To do this, take a B12 supplement or choose fortified foods (some soy products are fortified), or add B12-fortified nutritional yeast flakes to food. Not all nutritional yeast flakes contain B12, however so you need to check the pack.

MAKE DISCOVERIES

Be adventurous and try new and foreign foods. Many foods that might seem new to you may actually have a very long history in other parts of the world and sustained people for perhaps thousands of years. Antioxidant-rich cacao, protein-packed quinoa and omega-3-rich chia seeds, for example, are ancient foods from South America with healthy properties that have only recently been fully understood elsewhere.

In this book you'll find plenty of ways to use a variety of foods that are full of health benefits. Most are available from health-food stores and many can be bought in supermarkets. In the next section I list the foods to search out for keeping in stock, explain why they make healthy choices, how to use them and what to use as alternatives.

The Vegan Pantry

You can stock up your pantry gradually. I love to visit specialty stores, international delis and markets to buy spices, condiments and ingredients, and then make a dish taste new by adding a different spice or flavoring from my growing selection.

To save costs, I buy a lot of my legumes (peas, beans and lentils) in bulk, as well as almonds and cashews to make "milks" and raw desserts. (You could also share a bulk buy with a friend.) For taste and health reasons, everything I eat is organic, and I recommend you do the same. I stock up with fresh, organic fruit and vegetables at least once a week.

Most of the ingredients in this book are easy to find and you can substitute the more unusual ones with readily available alternatives. I have chosen to use healthy ingredients in this cookbook, because these are what I eat. You'll still be able to make most of the recipes without them though. The more exotic ingredients can usually be found at a well-stocked health-food store, and all can be purchased from online suppliers, if necessary.

Some of the foods listed below may be unfamiliar, but are chosen for their health benefits. Alternatives are given, but where possible, gradually try to increase the healthier versions in your own pantry. As mentioned earlier, I choose to limit my soy intake. Soy is found in many things, not just soy milk, and is often labeled as lecithin (soy based), hydrolyzed soy protein (HSP), MSG (monosodium glutamate), mono- and di-glycerides, among others.

Almonds High in magnesium, vitamin E, phosphorus and calcium, almonds are a great convenience snack and they make incredible milk.
Antipasti vegetables Sun-dried tomatoes and artichokes stored in oil in jars (or artichokes in brine from a can), are handy to add to a tomato-based pasta sauce for a quick and easy dinner or to serve on a platter with vegan cheese and biscuits.
Cacao nibs are shelled and crushed cacao beans. They have a dark, bitter taste, and a small amount will add a chocolatey flavor to any dish. This is *real*, unprocessed chocolate, containing feel-good nutrients

such as theobromine, phenylethylamine and anandamide. If you don't have raw cacao nibs or raw cacao powder, a high-quality vegan dark chocolate will suffice.

Cacao powder is made from raw, ground cacao beans and has a fairly bitter, rich and earthy taste. Rich in magnesium and antioxidants, it is a healthier choice than cocoa, which is highly processed and has lost much of the nutritional value that was present in the raw product. You can use cocoa instead of cacao, but not if you are making a raw recipe.

Canned/packaged foods Where possible, choose organic versions of tomato sauce, canned tomatoes and legumes. Avoid cans that are lined with the toxic plastic bisphenol A (BPA).

Carob powder Carob, a legume (bean), has a mildly sweet and fruity taste. Unlike chocolate, it contains no caffeine. The powder can be used in place of cacao or cocoa in recipes. Milder-flavored raw carob has not been heat treated and is preferable for raw desserts.

Chia seeds are ancient Mexican seeds that have recently been gaining recognition because of their healthy properties. They are high in the essential fatty acids, omega-3 and -6, and they are useful for vegans because they contain vital omega-3, which is difficult to obtain from animal-free sources. Chia seeds can be added to smoothies, cereals, baked products, soups and salads. They also make an egg replacer for binding by soaking in 1 or 2 tablespoons water until they form a gel.

Coconut aminos is similar to soy sauce, but without the soy. It is less salty, but it still has the same kick you expect from soy sauce or tamari. It can be used in place of both.

Coconut cream is the thick, solid layer that forms on the top of coconut milk, if the fat content is high enough, and is also sold as cream in cartons and cans. For extra-thick cream, store the carton or can upright in the refrigerator, then open it and take off the cream from the top.

Coconut milk is a more liquid equivalent of coconut cream. The thickness and quality of milk varies according to the brand. I choose cream most of the time and water it down myself if I need milk.

Coconut nectar is a mineral-rich liquid from the sap of coconut trees.

It has a caramel-butterscotch flavor and can be used in place of honey, agave syrup, and any plain sugar product. It has a low GI, and it also contains vitamin C.

Coconut oil has a fairly high smoke point (350°F), and so is suitable for frying. It can be heated without being damaged and oxidized, as other oils are. Oxidation causes oils to become unhealthy free radicals in the body. Choose organic, virgin and unrefined coconut oil, which is minimally processed. Non-virgin coconut oil may be produced from dried coconut (copra) and will have lost nutrients as well as being highly processed. Use coconut oil for baking, frying and in desserts or smoothies.

Alternatively, use OLIVE OIL (not extra virgin) for frying over medium heat. Organic SAFFLOWER OIL is high in omega-6 essential fats and is my personal alternative for cooking if I am short of coconut oil. RICE BRAN OIL is rich in vitamin E and omega-6, and has a high smoke point at 450°F. The only oil suitable for raw dishes, however, is coconut oil—for taste, nutrition and its ability to solidify quickly.

Coconut sugar Compared to cane sugar, coconut sugar has a lower GI. It is also rich in minerals and its mild caramel taste makes it a good alternative to cane sugar. You can make the recipes in this book using brown sugar, but do try to find coconut sugar to make sweet dishes healthier if you can. Coconut sugar is classed as raw, so it is used instead of brown sugar for recipes in this book that are labeled as raw. AGAVE SYRUP is sometimes given as a sweetener, although I rarely use it because it is high in fructose, which can lead to weight gain. BROWN RICE SYRUP is my preferred alternative as a sweetening syrup.

Coconut yogurt A relative newcomer to the market, dairy-free coconut yogurt is a wonderful substitute for soy yogurt. It is rich and creamy and has the most amazing taste. Store it in the refrigerator.

Dried fruits Providing they are organic and sulfur-free, dried fruits, such as cherries, cranberries, apricots and dates, can be used in a number of dishes. (See also Medjool dates, below.)

Gluten-free flour is available in a variety of types, such as brown rice, coconut, buckwheat and gram (chickpea). Your local health-food store or supermarket should stock a range, and you can also buy gluten-free flour blends, although these vary in quality. All gluten-free flours work slightly differently from regular flour and I recommend you try different ones to see which you prefer. Coconut flour is a tricky ingredient to work with because it absorbs a lot of liquid. If you try it, use only 20 to 30 percent of the quantity of the regular flour stated in the recipe.

Goji berries These nutrient-rich fruits can taste both tart and sweet. Use them in smoothies, salads, raw desserts and curries.

Grains Whole grains contain fiber and minerals that are lost when grains are processed. Use grains such as quinoa, brown rice and polenta, in place of white pasta. Quinoa and brown rice are also good for bulking up soups, salads and even breakfasts.

Green super-foods include SPIRULINA—a green sea algae that is high in protein and vitamins—and BARLEY GRASS/WHEATGRASS—a highly alkalizing product that can help balance the acid/alkaline levels in the body. They are not essential for the recipes and are quite pricey, but I feel they benefit my energy, skin and eyes.

Legumes The high protein content of legumes makes them important in the vegan diet. They are also rich in amino acids—the body's building blocks. Lentils, kidney beans, chickpeas, fava beans and lima beans are legumes that are cheap to buy, convenient to use and make a dish filling and sustaining. Dried red lentils cook in just 20 minutes, and many other legumes can be bought ready-cooked in cans.

Maca is a Peruvian root that may balance hormones. It has a fruity taste and can be added to raw desserts, smoothies and hot drinks.

Medjool dates Dates are high in fiber and a natural sweetener, which makes them useful to add to smoothies and raw desserts instead of using sugar or a syrup. I use fresh medjool dates in recipes because they are large and soft, but you can use dried dates, although sometimes you may need to soak them first.

Miso is a fermented soy product, also containing rice or barley, and can be beneficial to the digestion. Miso is salty and makes a great base for soups and Asian dishes. You can store dried miso in your cupboard, but miso paste should be stored in the refrigerator.

Nut butters Raw nut butters are a delicious, fresh alternative to regular store-bought peanut butter. You can make them yourself if you have a powerful blender. Almond butter, cashew butter and pecan butter are my favorites, but you can also make butters with macadamias, hazelnuts and walnuts. Use them as you would regular peanut butter, add them to smoothies and raw desserts or eat straight from the jar.

Nuts are a great way to get protein into a vegan diet (don't be scared by the fat content). They contain healthy fats when eaten raw and unprocessed. You can add a variety to your diet, such as almonds, macadamias, hazelnuts, pecans and pistachios, walnuts and peanuts (which are actually a legume, although we still eat them as a nut). Eat them alone, in salads, soups and stews, in raw desserts and smoothies, or blend them into nut butters.

Nutritional yeast flakes have a cheesy flavor and are bright yellow in color. Add them to soups, stews or pasta, or use them to make a vegan cheese sauce (page 23). They contain B vitamins, and some brands are high in essential B12, a bacterium found easily in animal products, so are useful for vegans.

Olives Add black or green olives to pasta, salads and antipasti for a delicious salty kick.

Seaweeds are rich in iodine and offer a broad range of other nutrients: B vitamins, folate, magnesium, iron, calcium and riboflavin. Salty-flavored NORI sheets are used to make sushi. AGAR-AGAR is used to set jellos and desserts in a similar way to the animal product, gelatin.

Seeds High in protein and minerals, sesame, pumpkin, sunflower and flaxseeds are just a few of the healthy seeds available. You can sprinkle them on salads and soups, and make them into milks.

Shredded coconut and coconut flakes are nutritious and useful for adding to cakes, muffins and smoothies.

Soy products Soy is a good way for vegans to get protein into their diets, but look for non-GM and organic brands. TOFU can be used in savory and sweet dishes due to its bland taste and color, and its ability to absorb other flavors. TEMPEH is a nutty-tasting fermented soy product, which needs to be cooked before eating.

Soy sauces Salty-flavored soy sauce and tamari are made from fermented soy beans. TAMARI is gluten-free, and both can be used interchangeably in many recipes.

Tahini, made from sesame seeds, is protein-rich and, when raw, is high in vitamins E, B1 B2 and A.

SPICES AND FLAVORINGS

Good basics for spicy dishes include dried cumin, coriander, turmeric and cinnamon, plus dried and crushed chilies, and also always have some fresh chilies in the refrigerator. For an authentic touch, try:

Chermoula paste A mixture of herbs, spices, oil and lemon used in Moroccan dishes. Add it to tagines or to vegetables before roasting.

Galangal A root with an aromatic, peppery flavor.

Garam masala A mixture of Indian spices, predominantly cinnamon, cumin, peppercorns, cloves and cardamom.

Harissa A hot and spicy chili paste used in North African cooking.

Kaffir lime leaves, which lend a tang and fragrance to Thai cooking. Freeze fresh leaves up to 8 months in a freezer bag.

Lemongrass to give Thai and Asian cooking that distinctive flavor. Buy it fresh and store it in the refrigerator.

Mirin A low-alcohol Japanese rice wine, with a sweet "kick." It can transform the flavor of a stir-fry.

Paprika, either sweet or smoked, adds a deep level of flavor and aroma to dishes, particularly those from Mexico and Morocco.

Rice wine vinegar to add depth of flavor to Asian dishes.

Tamarind is used in Asian cooking for its sweet, sour and tangy flavor.

Vanilla The seeds of vanilla beans are used widely in this book. Use the pods to flavor sugar. Vanilla bean paste is a convenient way to get the flavor of vanilla from a bean without the effort.

You can also use cashews, macadamias, hazelnuts or sesame seeds to create your own dairy-free milks.

almond milk

Makes: 3¼ cups
Preparation: 15 minutes,
  plus overnight soaking

1 cup almonds with skins

OPTIONAL
1 vanilla bean
2 fresh or dried medjool
  dates, pitted

Put the almonds in a bowl, cover with water and let soak overnight. Drain in a colander and rinse well, then drain again. If using the vanilla bean, split the bean in half lengthwise and scrape out the seeds. Reserve the bean for another use.

Put the almonds into a blender or food processor with 2 cups water and the vanilla seeds and dates, if using. Blend on high speed 1 to 2 minutes. Check the consistency. If you prefer your milk thinner, add up to 1 cup water and pulse to combine.

Strain through a nut-milk bag, or a fine strainer, muslin or cheesecloth. (The almonds can be drip-dried for a wetter pulp—perfect for making cheese. Place the bag filled with pulp onto an upturned saucer inside a larger bowl and put a heavy weight, such as a can of beans, on a small plate on top of the bag.)

Reserve the pulp for later use (see Herbed Almond Cheese, page 22). The milk can be stored in a sealed glass jar in the refrigerator up to 4 days and can also be frozen in icecube trays, and the cubes stored in freezer bags up to 2 months.

   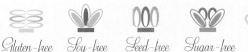

Gluten-free   *Soy-free*   *Seed-free*   *Sugar-free*   *Raw*

white cottage-feta cheese

Makes: 1 cup
Preparation: 20 minutes, plus
  overnight soaking and an
  optional overnight pressing

1 cup macadamias
¼ cup pitted green olives,
  chopped
1 teaspoon grated lemon zest
juice of 1 lemon
½ teaspoon crushed chilies
  (optional)
¼ teaspoon freshly ground
  black pepper
sea salt

Put the macadamias in a bowl, cover with water and let soak overnight. Drain in a colander, then rinse well and drain again.

Put the macadamias into a blender or food processor with ½ cup water. Blend into a fine paste. Using a nut-milk bag, or a fine strainer, muslin or cheesecloth, squeeze out the excess water.

Stir in the olives, lemon zest and juice, crushed chilies, if using, and pepper, then add salt to taste. The cheese should be white, with a cottage-cheese consistency, but it should be salty like feta. The cheese is ready to eat right away or it can be pressed to make it firm. To do this, wrap the cheese in muslin or cheesecloth and put it on a plate. Put a heavy weight, such as a can of beans, on a small plate on top of the cheese and leave overnight.

Gluten-free

Soy-free

Seed-free

Sugar-free

Raw

You can use leftover Almond Milk pulp (page 20) here, but without soaking and processing the almonds. Vary the herbs, if you like (but don't add the onion and garlic if using cilantro), or use 2 chopped chilies, 1½ tablespoons ground black pepper or ⅔ cup chopped ready-to-eat dried apricots. Try rolling the cheese in herbs or coarsely ground peppercorns.

herbed almond cheese

Makes: 1 pound, 2 ounces
Preparation: 25 minutes, plus
   overnight soaking, 4 hours
   fermenting, 3 hours chilling

2⅓ cups almonds with skins
½ red onion, chopped
1 garlic clove, crushed
1 teaspoon lemon juice
1 small handful of parsley
   leaves, finely chopped
2 teaspoons miso
1 tablespoon finely chopped
   dill
freshly ground black pepper

Put the almonds in a bowl, cover with water and let soak overnight. Drain in a colander, then rinse well and drain again. If you like, you can remove the skins by rubbing them with a dry dish towel. (If you remove the skins you will have a sweeter-flavored cheese.)

Put the almonds into a blender or food processor and add 1 cup water. Blend until smooth and then strain through a nut-milk bag, or a fine strainer, muslin or cheesecloth.

Roll the pulp into a ball and put it back into the nut-milk bag, then put the bag in a bowl. Put a heavy weight, such as a can of beans, on a small plate on top of the bag of pulp and let it ferment 3 to 4 hours.

Put the strained almond pulp back into the blender, and add the onion, garlic and lemon juice. Season with pepper, then blend until well combined. Tip into a bowl and add the parsley, miso and dill. Mix well, then roll into a ball. Chill in the refrigerator 3 hours before serving.

Gluten-free   *Seed-free*   *Sugar-free*   *Raw*

Nutritional yeast flakes give this savory sauce a rich, cheese-like flavor. Use the sauce in lasagne, with pasta or as a dip for lightly steamed vegetables.

vegan cheese sauce

Makes: about 2⅓ cups
Preparation: 15 minutes,
   plus 30 minutes soaking
Cooking: 15 minutes

1 cup cashews
2 cups rice milk
1½ cups nutritional
   yeast flakes
1 teaspoon miso, soy sauce or
   tamari soy sauce
juice of ½ lemon
1 tablespoon rice flour or all-
   purpose flour
freshly ground black pepper

Put the cashews in a bowl, cover with water and let soak 30 minutes. Drain the cashews in a colander and put them into a blender or food processor, then blend until fine.

Pour the milk into a medium saucepan over medium heat and add 1 cup water. Whisk together and bring gently to a boil, then reduce the heat to a simmer.

Add the yeast flakes, ground cashews, miso, lemon juice and flour. Season with pepper and whisk until smooth. The sauce will thicken after a minute or so. Once thickened, remove from the heat and serve or use in your chosen recipe.

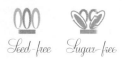

Seed-free   *Sugar-free*

Use this versatile, fresh tomato sauce as a base for a vegetable sauce with nuts, legumes or tempeh to serve over pasta or grains. Or serve it with polenta, pies or the Red Lentil & Beet Burgers (page 148) instead of the relish and buns.

tomato sauce

Makes: about 8½ cups
Preparation: 25 minutes
Cooking: 3½ hours

11 pounds plum tomatoes or other ripe tomatoes
1 tablespoon olive oil or safflower oil
1 garlic bulb, cloves crushed
4 onions, thinly sliced
1 handful of basil leaves, chopped
1 teaspoon brown sugar or coconut sugar, plus extra if needed
sea salt and freshly ground black pepper

Cut the tomatoes in half and cut out the cores, then roughly chop the flesh. Put the tomatoes in a pan over medium heat and cook 20 minutes, stirring occasionally, so that the tomatoes release their juice—they do not need any added water.

Heat the oil in a shallow saucepan over medium heat and cook the garlic and onions 5 to 8 minutes until softened.

Tip the onion mixture into the tomatoes and add the basil, then stir well. Using a blender or food processor, blend the mixture until smooth. You may have to do this in batches.

Add 1 teaspoon sugar and 1 teaspoon salt, then taste. If the sauce is too tart, add more sugar. If the sauce is too sweet, add more salt. Add pepper to taste.

Simmer the sauce over medium heat 3 hours, or until reduced and thick. Serve, or add to your recipe, or let cool. Once cold, the sauce can be transferred to sterilized jars and stored up to 4 days in the refrigerator or divided into 1 cup portions and frozen in freezer bags up to 2 months.

Gluten-free   Soy-free   Nut-free   Seed-free

Traditionally, this paste is pounded, ingredient by ingredient, using a mortar and pestle, but my faster version uses a blender. Use either red or green chilies to change the color and heat of the paste—Thai chilies have the best flavor.

thai red or green curry paste

Makes: about ½ cup
Preparation: 15 minutes
Cooking: 5 minutes

1 teaspoon coriander seeds
1 teaspoon white
  peppercorns
2 lemongrass stalks, outer
  leaves and stalk removed,
  white part only
3 shallots
10 garlic cloves
1-inch piece fresh ginger
  root, peeled
1-inch piece galangal,
  peeled, or ½-inch piece
  fresh ginger root, peeled
grated zest of 1 lime,
  preferably kaffir lime
5 to 10 hot red chilies,
  preferably Thai, or milder
  green chilies, tops trimmed
juice of 1 lime
1 large handful of cilantro
  roots, stems and leaves

Put the coriander seeds and white peppercorns in a small pan and toast over medium heat 3 minutes, shaking the pan frequently, to release the aroma. Remove from the heat.

Put all the ingredients into a blender or food processor and blend into a paste. Use immediately or store in the refrigerator up to 1 week. The paste can also be frozen in icecube trays and the cubes stored in freezer bags up to 2 months.

Gluten-free   Soy-free   Nut-free   Seed-free   Sugar-free

fruit & pumpkin spread

Makes: about 3 cups
Preparation: 20 minutes
Cooking: 1 hour 10 minutes

6 apricots or 3 peaches, cut
 in half and pitted
11 ounces pumpkin or
 butternut squash, peeled
 and cubed
4 large pears or apples,
 peeled, cored and cubed
1 cup brown sugar or
 coconut sugar
1 teaspoon ground cinnamon
½ teaspoon ground
 cardamom
½ teaspoon ground ginger
½ teaspoon ground allspice

Put all the ingredients in a large, heavy saucepan and add ¾ cup water, then combine well.

Bring to a boil over medium heat, then reduce the heat to low and simmer 1 hour, stirring frequently, or until the pumpkin and fruit are soft. Add extra water if the mixture starts to stick on the bottom of the pan. Pour the mixture into a blender or food processor and blend until smooth. Serve or cool and store in a covered container in the refrigerator up to 7 days.

Gluten-free Soy-free Nut-free Seed-free

chocolate & hazelnut butter

Makes: 2½ cups
Preparation: 10 minutes

1 vanilla bean
2 cups hazelnuts
⅓ cup raw cacao powder
⅓ cup brown rice syrup or
 agave syrup
a pinch of sea salt

Split the vanilla bean in half lengthwise and scrape out the seeds. Reserve the bean for another use. Put the seeds to one side. Put the hazelnuts in a blender or food processor and grind until smooth. Continue to grind until the nuts become butter. Add the cacao powder, syrup, vanilla seeds and salt. Pulse to combine. Serve or store in a sterilized jar in the refrigerator up to 2 weeks.

Gluten-free Soy-free Seed-free Raw

Homemade Indian breads are fast and easy to make, and they taste very good indeed. You can make them by hand or using a food processor while your curry is simmering.

garlic parathas

Makes: 8 parathas
Preparation: 20 minutes,
**   plus 10 minutes resting**
Cooking: 15 minutes

2 cups wholewheat flour, plus
    extra for dusting
2 tablespoons good-quality
    olive oil
a pinch of sea salt
2 garlic cloves, crushed

Preheat the oven to 200°F and put a heatproof plate inside to warm.

Sift the flour into a large bowl, tipping in any bran left in the sifter, and add the remaining ingredients and ½ cup lukewarm water. Stir well to combine thoroughly, then turn out onto a floured work surface. Knead 2 minutes, or until the dough is smooth and springy, and then put it in a floured bowl and set to one side to rest 10 minutes. (Alternatively, if you have a food processor with a kneading attachment, add all the ingredients and knead until the dough combines.)

Heat a nonstick skillet over medium heat. Divide the dough into 8 pieces and flatten them with your hands. Working carefully to retain the stretchy dough, flatten one piece with a rolling pin, then put it in the hot skillet. Cook 1 minute, then turn it over, using a spatula. Cook another 1 minute, then press down with a clean, dry dish towel to ensure the paratha cooks evenly.

Wrap the paratha in foil and keep warm in the oven while you cook the remaining dough, or serve each paratha as soon as it comes out of the skillet.

Soy-free   Nut-free   Seed-free   Sugar-free

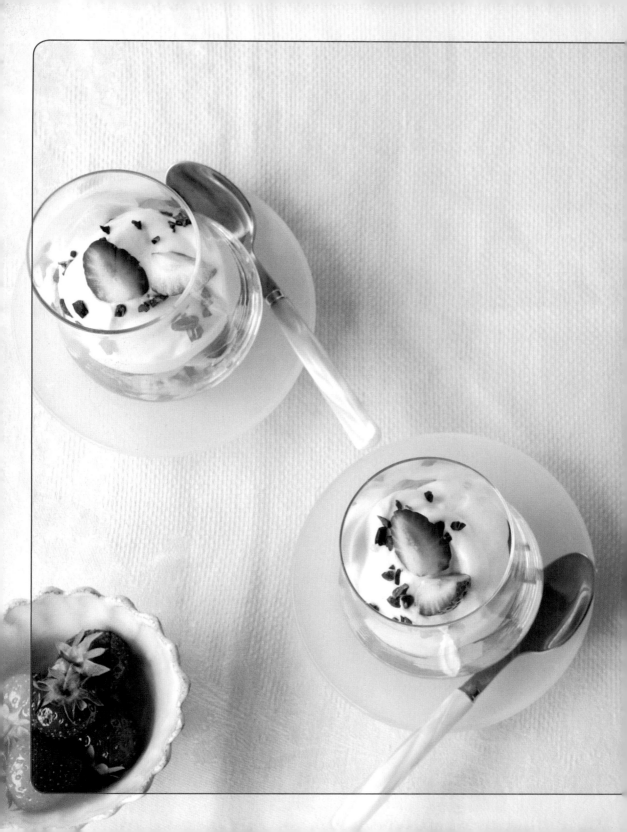

Breakfasts &
Brunches

Often called the most important meal of the day, breakfast should be nourishing and appealing with plenty of variety. There are tempting breakfasts here for every day of the week. Long brunches and lazy breakfasts can be on everyone's weekend menu, because all the recipes here are fast to prepare, and some can be left to cook slowly, such as the Breakfast Tagine, giving you maximum weekend relaxation with minimal effort. Weekdays are simple as well. You will find a smoothie to go, or a fruit salad with a twist. A Chocolate Mudslide Smoothie will kick-start your day, and my Watermelon & Orange Salad will freshen you up. Some breakfasts can even be made in advance—try Peanut Butter & Banana Bread, Tea-Poached Prunes or Toasted Granola. Throw some breakfast together and let the good days roll.

Over-the-Top Banana
Oatmeal (page 41).

peach passion smoothie

Serves: 2
Preparation: 10 minutes,
  plus making the milk

4 ripe peaches, cut into
  quarters and pitted
2 passionfruits, cut in half
  and flesh scooped out
2¾ cups Almond Milk
  (page 20)
1 large handful of ice cubes
1 fresh or dried medjool date,
  pitted
1 teaspoon coconut oil
  (optional)
fresh mint leaves, to serve

Put all the ingredients into a blender or food processor and blend at high speed until smooth and creamy. Serve in tall glasses and decorate with fresh mint leaves.

Gluten-free   *Soy-free*   *Seed-free*   *Sugar-free*   *Raw*

chocolate mudslide smoothie

Serves: 2
Preparation: 10 minutes,
  plus overnight freezing
  and making the milk

2 bananas, peeled and
  chopped
2 tablespoons raw cacao
  powder
1 tablespoon cacao nibs
1 tablespoon carob powder
2¾ cups Almond Milk
  (page 20)
1 teaspoon ground cinnamon
1 teaspoon maca powder
  (optional)
1 teaspoon spirulina
  (optional)
shredded coconut, to serve

Put the bananas in a freezer bag, seal and freeze overnight. The next day, put all the ingredients into a blender or food processor and blend at high speed until smooth and creamy. Top with shredded coconut to serve.

Gluten-free   *Soy-free*   *Seed-free*   *Sugar-free*   *Raw*

black forest *smoothie*

Serves: 2
Preparation: 10 minutes,
  plus making the milk

1 vanilla bean
3¼ cups Almond Milk
  (page 20)
1 cup fresh or frozen cherries,
  pitted
2 tablespoons raw cacao
  powder
1 tablespoon carob powder
1 tablespoon almond butter
1½ teaspoons ground
  cinnamon
2 fresh or dried medjool
  dates, pitted
1 tablespoon chia seeds

Split the vanilla bean in half lengthwise and scrape out the seeds. Reserve the bean for another use. Put the seeds into a blender or food processor and add the remaining ingredients. Blend until smooth and creamy, then serve immediately.

Gluten-free Soy-free Sugar-free Raw

cucumber, lime & *watermelon juice*

Serves: 2
Preparation: 10 minutes

2 cucumbers, cut into
  quarters
1 lime, peeled and cut into
  quarters
1¼ pounds watermelon,
  roughly chopped
1 handful of fresh mint
  leaves, chopped
ice cubes, to serve

Put the cucumbers, lime and watermelon through an electric juicer. Add the mint and serve over ice. (Alternatively, juice the mint with the other ingredients, if you like.)

Gluten-free Soy-free Nut-free Seed-free Sugar-free Raw

The cooling and sweet watermelon in this breakfast salad is set off by tangy orange and lime. It's high in soluble fiber, antioxidants and vitamin C, as well as beta-carotene and potassium, making it a perfect way to start the day.

watermelon & *orange salad*

Serves: 2
Preparation: 15 minutes,
   plus 30 minutes chilling

1 orange
1¼ pounds watermelon,
   cut into slices
1 small cucumber, cut in half
   and thinly sliced
2 tablespoons lime juice
1 tablespoon mint leaves
grated zest of 1 lime
dairy-free yogurt, to serve
   (optional)

Using a sharp knife, cut a thin slice of peel and pith from each end of the orange. Put the orange cut-side down on a plate and cut off the peel and pith in strips. Remove any remaining pith. Cut out each segment, leaving the membrane behind.

Put the orange in a serving bowl, then squeeze in the remaining juice from the membrane. Add the watermelon, cucumber, lime juice and mint, then toss together. Sprinkle with lime zest, then cover and chill in the refrigerator 30 minutes to allow the flavors to develop. Serve with dairy-free yogurt, if you like.

Gluten-free

Soy-free

Nut-free

Seed-free

Sugar-free

Raw

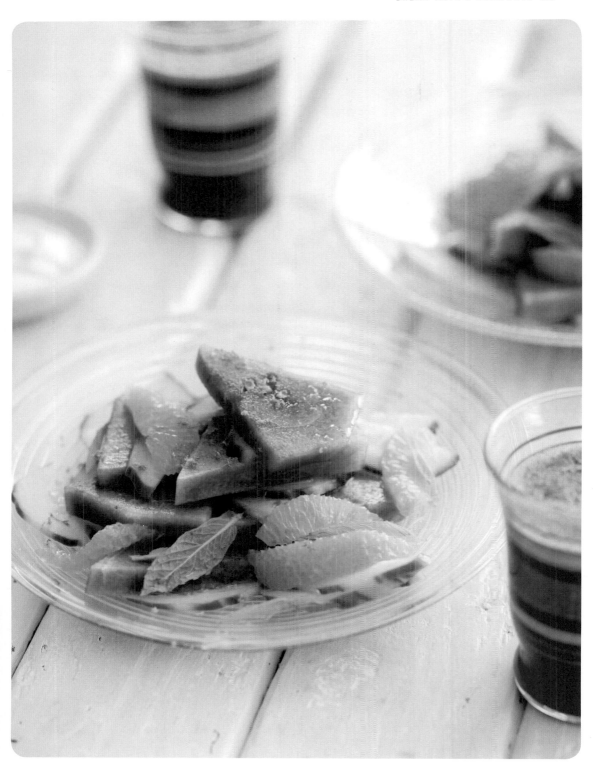

In this recipe, the sweetness of the prunes is offset by the floral bergamot and tannins from the Earl Grey tea they are poached in. This is a simple breakfast that can be prepared the night before—and it keeps for a few days.

tea-poached *prunes*

Serves: 6
Preparation: 5 minutes,
  plus overnight chilling
  and making the granola

2 cups ready-to-eat pitted
  prunes
½ cup orange juice
2 cups freshly brewed Earl
  Grey tea or English tea
Toasted Granola (page 36)
  and dairy-free yogurt,
  to serve

Put the prunes in a bowl and pour the orange juice and tea over them. Set to one side to cool, then cover and chill in the refrigerator overnight.

To serve, spoon the prunes and tea syrup over the granola and top with a spoonful of yogurt. Store the soaked prunes in a covered container in the refrigerator up to 4 days.

Gluten-free   Soy-free   Nut-free   Seed-free   Sugar-free

The options are endless for added toppings to this banana breakfast or dessert—hazelnuts, cranberries, fresh strawberries or raspberries and sliced oranges to name just a few, apart from the selection below. You can also make this into a smoothie by blending everything together, including the liquid from the carton of coconut cream.

banana split with coconut cream whip

Serves: 2
**Preparation: 15 minutes,
   plus overnight chilling**

1 cup coconut cream in the unopened carton or can
2 bananas
1 teaspoon vanilla paste or vanilla extract
1 tablespoon cacao nibs or chopped dark vegan chocolate
1 tablespoon goji berries or dried cranberries
1 tablespoon slivered almonds
1 teaspoon pumpkin seeds
1 teaspoon sunflower seeds
1 teaspoon carob powder, cocoa powder or raw cacao powder
1 teaspoon ground cinnamon

Chill the coconut cream overnight in the refrigerator, making sure the carton is upright. Without shaking the carton, open it and scoop off the cream from the top. It will be very, very thick. Put the cream into a blender or food processor and set the coconut liquid to one side

Peel the bananas and cut them in half lengthwise, then put two halves in each of two serving bowls.

Add the vanilla to the blender. Pour in some of the reserved coconut liquid, 1 tablespoon at a time, while blending 2 to 3 minutes until the coconut cream is soft but thick enough to hold its shape. Spoon onto the split bananas, and top with the cacao nibs, goji berries, almonds, and pumpkin and sunflower seeds. Dust with carob powder and cinnamon, then serve.

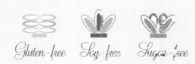

Gluten-free   Soy-free   Sugar-free

Soy-free

toasted *granola*

Serves: 6
Preparation: 15 minutes,
  plus making the milk
  and optional prunes
Cooking: 20 minutes,
  plus cooling

2⅔ cups rolled oats
2 cups seed and grain
  mix (sesame, pumpkin,
  sunflower, rye, barley, bran)
1 cup almonds, chopped
1 cup pecans, roughly
  chopped
½ cup safflower oil, sunflower
  oil or melted coconut oil
¼ cup brown sugar or
  coconut sugar
2 teaspoons ground
  cinnamon
Almond Milk (page 20) and
  fresh fruit, or Tea-Poached
  Prunes (page 34), to serve

Preheat the oven to 315°F and line a baking tray with baking parchment. Put the oats in a large bowl and add the seed and grain mixture, almonds and pecans.

Put the oil in a small bowl and add the sugar and cinnamon. Whisk together, then drizzle it over the oat mixture. Stir well to ensure the oat mixture is thoroughly coated. Spread out evenly on the prepared baking tray and bake 10 minutes, then shake the mixture and bake another 10 minutes. Let cool, then serve with almond milk and fresh fruit. Store in a sterilized glass jar, in a cool dry place, up to 3 weeks.

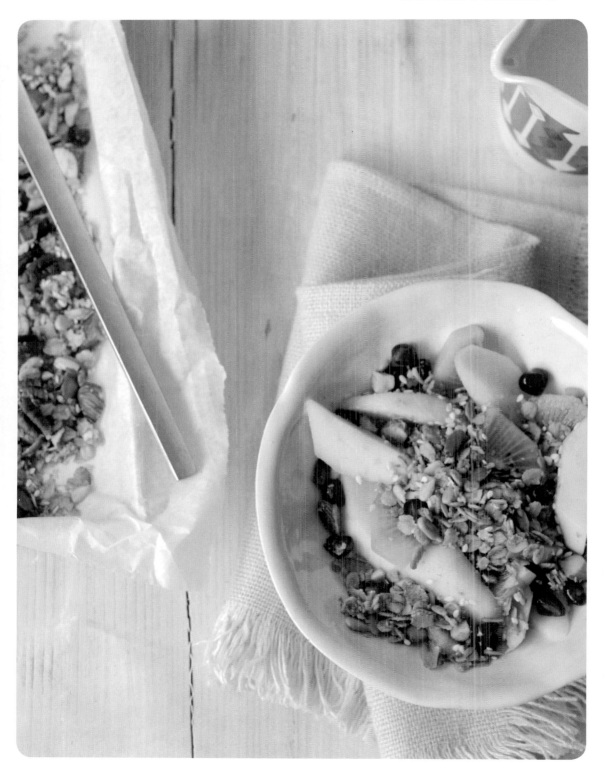

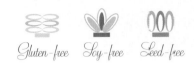

Gluten-free   Soy-free   Seed-free

quinoa porridge with rhubarb & *apple compote*

Serves: 2 (with compote left over)
Preparation: 15 minutes, plus cooling and making the milk
Cooking: 40 minutes

½ cup plus 1½ tablespoons quinoa, rinsed and drained
2 cups Almond Milk (page 20), plus extra to serve
1 tablespoon brown sugar or coconut sugar
1 tablespoon vanilla extract
1 teaspoon ground cinnamon

RHUBARB AND APPLE COMPOTE
1 pound rhubarb, chopped
2 apples, peeled, cored and chopped
⅓ cup brown sugar or coconut sugar

To make the compote, put all the ingredients in a medium saucepan and add ½ cup water. Combine well and bring to a boil over medium heat, then reduce the heat to low. Make sure that the rhubarb and apples are completely submerged. Stir to dissolve the sugar. Simmer 10 to 15 minutes, until the rhubarb is soft.

Let the compote cool completely, then pour into a sterilized glass jar. Store in the refrigerator 1 week, or divide into portions in freezer bags and freeze up to 1 month.

To make the porridge, put the quinoa in a heavy saucepan and add the milk, sugar, vanilla and cinnamon. Stir well to combine, then bring to a gentle boil over medium heat. Cook 20 minutes, stirring occasionally, or until the quinoa is tender and translucent and the porridge has thickened. Serve with a dash of milk, and some of the compote. (The compote can also be served with ice cream, in smoothies or spread on pancakes.)

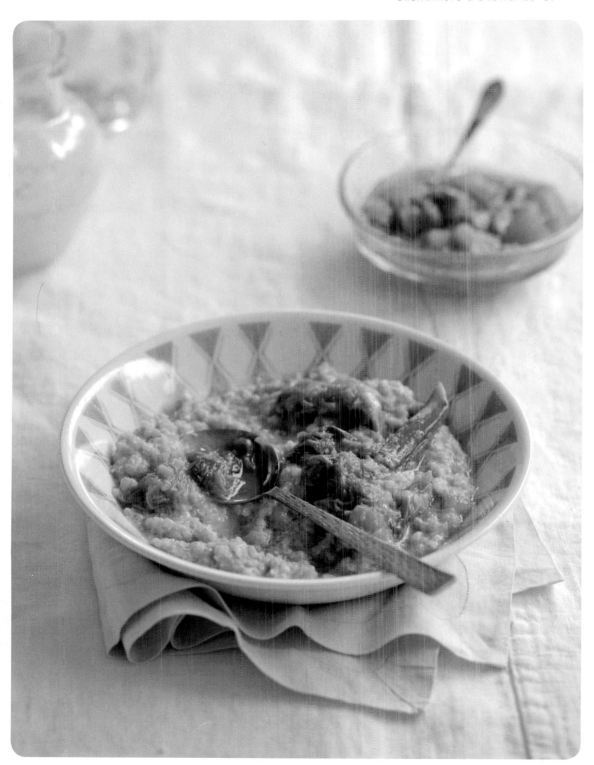

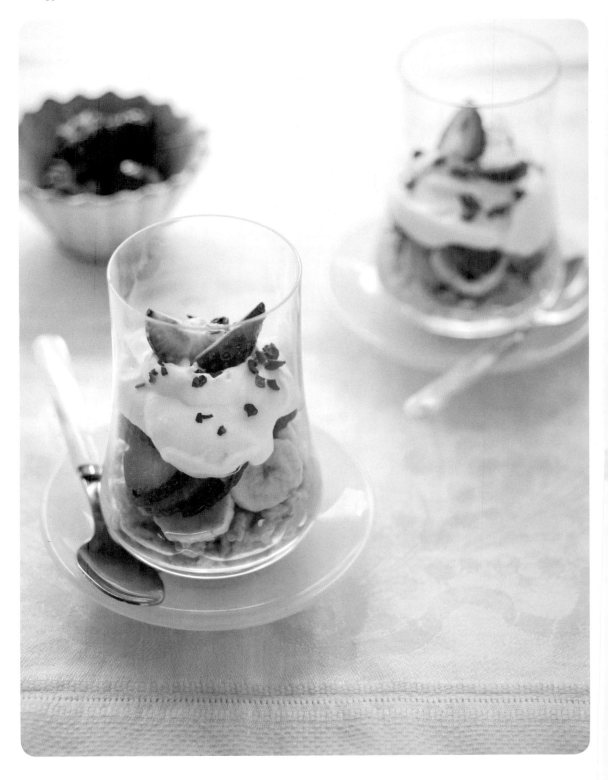

Served in a tall glass, this looks more like a dessert than a breakfast. The oatmeal can be made the night before. If you like, add some chia seeds to your yogurt to include some healthy omega-3 and -6 fats, plus more fiber and protein.

over-the-top banana *oatmeal*

Serves: 2
Preparation: 20 minutes,
  plus cooling and 1 hour
  or overnight chilling,
  and making the milk
Cooking: 20 minutes

⅔ cup rolled oats
1½ cups Almond Milk
  (page 20)
1 teaspoon brown sugar or
  coconut sugar
½ teaspoon ground
  cinnamon, plus extra
  to serve
a pinch of sea salt
1 banana, thinly sliced
9 ounces (about 2½ cups)
  strawberries, hulled and
  sliced
1 cup dairy-free coconut
  yogurt
2 tablespoons cacao nibs or
  vegan chocolate chips
carob powder, cocoa powder
  or raw cacao powder
  (optional), to serve

Put the oats in a medium saucepan and add the milk, ½ cup water, the sugar, cinnamon and salt.

Bring to a gentle boil over medium heat, then reduce the heat to a simmer and cook 10 minutes, stirring frequently. Add a little more water if the mixture is too thick. Cook another 5 minutes, or until thickened like porridge. Remove from the heat, then cool and chill in the refrigerator 1 hour or overnight.

Spoon some oatmeal into two tall glasses, then add some banana slices, a few strawberry slices, and 1 tablespoon yogurt. Sprinkle with a few cacao nibs, then continue to layer until the glass is full. Top with any remaining strawberries and cacao nibs, dust with carob powder, if using, then serve. (Alternatively, make single layers, if you are using a larger glass.)

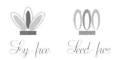
Soy-free   Seed-free

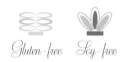

Gluten-free   Soy-free

chia seed & coconut *pancakes*

Serves: 4
Preparation: 30 minutes,
 plus 10 minutes soaking,
 plus making the spread
Cooking: 20 minutes

½ teaspoon chia seeds
1½ cups buckwheat flour
2 teaspoons gluten-free
 baking powder
3¾ cups coconut milk
½ cup Fruit & Pumpkin
 Spread (page 26), plus extra
 to serve
2 tablespoons olive oil,
 safflower oil or coconut oil,
 plus extra if needed
shredded coconut, berries,
 and agave syrup or brown
 rice syrup (optional),
 to serve

Preheat the oven to 200°F and put a heatproof plate inside to warm. Put the chia seeds in a small bowl and add 3 tablespoons water. Let soak 10 minutes to form a gel.

Sift the buckwheat flour and baking powder into a large mixing bowl and mix well.

In a separate bowl, whisk together the chia seed gel, coconut milk and the fruit spread. Add to the dry ingredients and stir gently to form a thick batter.

Heat 1½ teaspoons of the oil in a heavy skillet over medium heat. Pour 3 to 4 tablespoonfuls of batter into the pan, tilting the pan to cover the bottom of the pan with the mixture. Cook 2 to 3 minutes on each side until lightly browned.

Repeat with the remaining batter, adding another 1½ teaspoons oil to the pan before cooking each one. Transfer the pancakes to the warmed plate, stacking them between sheets of baking parchment to prevent them from sticking together, and keep warm in the oven. Serve hot with a selection of toppings.

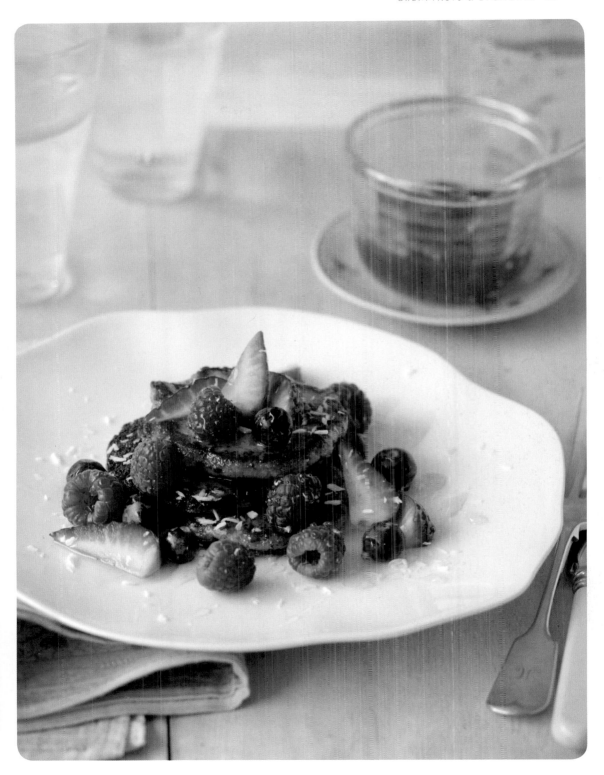

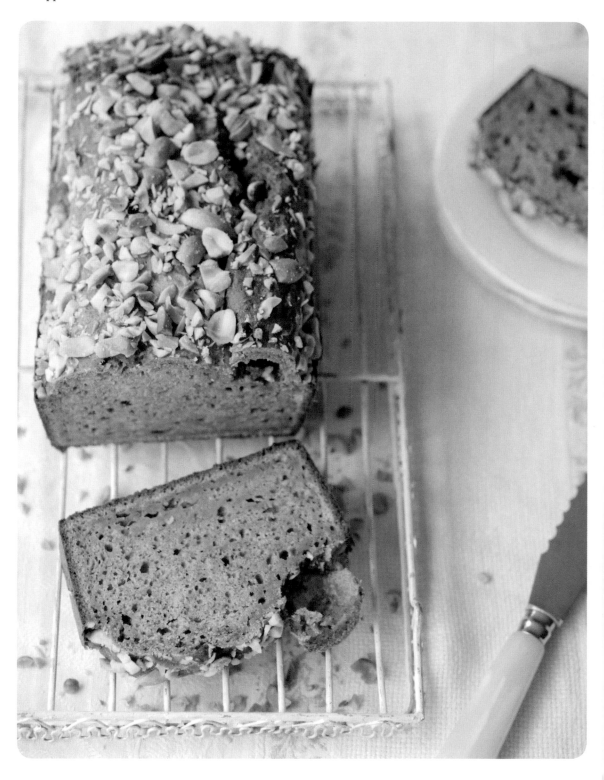

Banana makes this bread moist and flavorsome, and the peanuts add crunch and richness. You could also make the recipe using almond butter and even add some vegan chocolate chips.

peanut butter & banana bread

Makes: 1 loaf, 10 slices
Preparation: 15 minutes,
plus making the milk
Cooking: 45 minutes, plus
cooling

2 cups all-purpose flour
1½ teaspoons baking powder
1 vanilla bean
4 overripe bananas, cut into pieces
½ cup Almond Milk (page 20)
⅔ cup sugar-free crunchy peanut butter
¼ cup safflower oil, sunflower oil or melted coconut oil
1 teaspoon ground cinnamon
½ cup peanuts, roughly chopped

Preheat the oven to 350°F. Line the bottom and short sides of a nonstick 9 × 4-inch loaf pan with a strip of baking parchment and set aside. Sift the flour and baking powder into a large mixing bowl.

Split the vanilla bean in half lengthwise and scrape out the seeds. Reserve the bean for another use. Put the bananas in a separate bowl and add the milk, vanilla seeds, peanut butter, oil and cinnamon. Using a hand blender, combine the ingredients until they form a smooth batter.

Pour this mixture into the dry ingredients and fold gently to combine. Spoon the mixture into the prepared loaf pan and spread out evenly. Sprinkle the peanuts over the top. Bake 35 to 45 minutes until a skewer inserted into the center comes out clean. Transfer to a wire rack and let cool in the pan before removing and serving. Store in an airtight container up to 4 days.

Soy-free

Sugar-free

Sugar-free

cinnamon *crumpets*

Makes 6 crumpets
Preparation: 15 minutes, plus
 1 hour rising, and making
 the milk and optional butter
Cooking: 20 minutes

2 cups all-purpose flour
1 teaspoon ground cinnamon
½ teaspoon baking powder
a pinch of sea salt
¼-ounce envelope
 (2¾ teaspoons) fast-action
 dry yeast
¾ cup Almond Milk (page
 20), at room temperature
1 tablespoon vegan
 margarine, plus extra for
 frying
Chocolate & Hazelnut Butter
 (page 26) and fresh fruit
 (optional), to serve

Sift the flour, cinnamon, baking powder and salt into a large bowl. Add the yeast, milk, margarine and ½ cup water, at room temperature. Whisk, or use an electric blender, to combine the mixture until smooth. Cover the bowl, and leave in a warm place 1 hour, or until bubbles appear.

Put a small pat of margarine in a heavy, nonstick skillet over medium heat. Put two 4-inch nonstick metal food rings into the pan. Pour ¼ cup of the batter into each ring. Cook over medium heat 3 to 4 minutes until the batter comes away from the rings—you will see it firming up on the side of the ring.

Remove the food rings carefully, using tongs, and turn the crumpets over using a spatula. Cook the crumpets another 3 to 5 minutes until golden brown. (Alternatively, you can make the crumpets without the rings but they will be a pancake shape and will take less time to cook, 2 to 3 minutes on each side.) Wrap the crumpets in a clean dish towel and keep them warm, or serve them as you make them. Cook the remaining batter in the same way. Spread generously with the chocolate and hazelnut butter, and serve with some fresh fruit, if you like.

For extra protein you can add some silken tofu to this sustaining savory breakfast a few minutes before it has finished cooking, if you like.

greek breakfast scramble

Serves: 2
Preparation: 15 minutes
Cooking: 50 minutes

4 medium potatoes, cubed
1 tablespoon olive oil or rice
  bran oil
1 large onion, finely chopped
juice of 1½ lemons
½ red bell pepper, seeded
  and sliced
1½ cups button
  mushrooms, sliced
1 cup pitted Kalamata olives
1 small handful flat-leaf
  parsley leaves, torn
¼ cup finely chopped
  basil leaves
1 teaspoon finely shredded
  mint leaves
sliced avocado and cherry
  tomatoes, to serve

Put the potato cubes in a saucepan, cover well with boiling water and cook 5 to 8 minutes until just tender. Drain in a colander and set to one side.

Heat the oil in a heavy skillet over medium heat. Add the onion, and cook 10 minutes, or until translucent. Add the potatoes and lemon juice, and bring to a high simmer. Cook 15 minutes, or until the lemon juice has reduced and the potatoes are golden brown.

Add the pepper, mushrooms and olives, and cook 10 minutes. Remove from the heat and serve scattered with the parsley, basil and mint, and with the avocado slices and cherry tomatoes.

Gluten-free *Soy-free* *Nut-free* *Seed-free* *Sugar-free*

48

This versatile hash mixture can also be made into burgers or a rosti. Soak 1 tablespoon chia seeds in 3 tablespoons water 10 minutes, then stir into the cooked hash. Form into burger shapes and fry 5 minutes in a little oil.

sweet potato hash with tomato relish

Serves: 2 (with relish left over)
Preparation: 25 minutes
Cooking: 1 hour 10 minutes,
  plus cooling

1 tablespoon olive oil or
  coconut oil
9 ounces sweet potato, grated
1 large onion, chopped
2¼ ounces kale, thinly sliced
1 tablespoon lemon juice
chopped parsley leaves and
  cubed avocado, to serve

TOMATO RELISH
4 medium tomatoes, chopped
1 large onion, chopped
1 red bell pepper, seeded
  and cubed
1 teaspoon cider vinegar
2 teaspoons brown sugar or
  coconut sugar
1 teaspoon crushed chilies
1½ cups vegetable stock
sea salt and freshly ground
  black pepper

To make the relish, put all the ingredients in a large, heavy saucepan. Bring to a gentle boil over medium heat, then reduce the heat to a low simmer and cook 45 minutes, stirring frequently, or until the pepper is soft and the liquid has reduced. Adjust the seasoning to taste.

When the relish has thickened, remove the pan from the heat and let cool. Pour into a sterilized glass jar and store in the refrigerator up to 4 weeks.

To make the hash, heat the oil in a heavy skillet over medium heat and add the sweet potato and onion. Season with salt and pepper. Cook 10 minutes, stirring frequently, then add the kale and cook another 10 minutes, or until the sweet potato is crispy and the onion is soft. Drizzle the lemon juice over it and sprinkle with parsley. Serve with cubed avocado, and top with a large spoonful of tomato relish.

Gluten-free   *Soy-free*   *Nut-free*   *Seed-free*

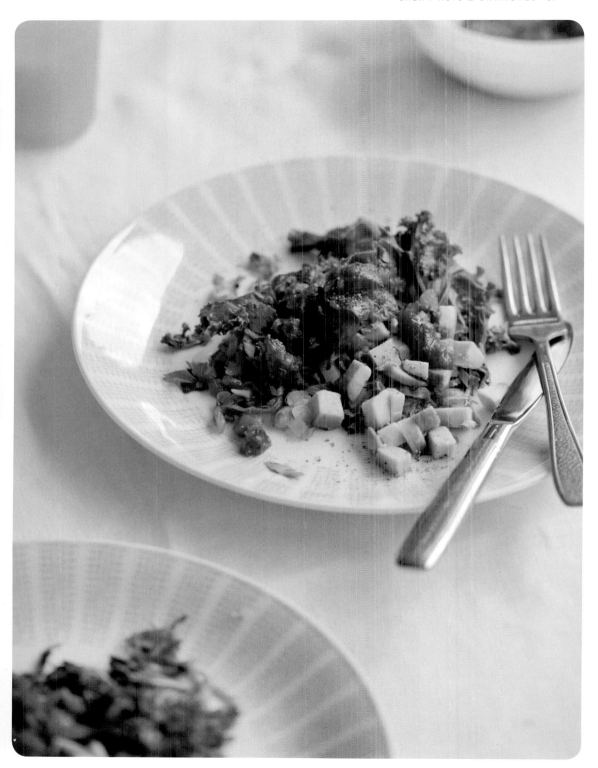

This is a sublimely easy dish that is perfect for those days when you feel like being really lazy and having an effortless breakfast. Add the ingredients to a casserole dish, pop it in the oven and leave it to cook, then come back later and enjoy! It can also be prepared and cooked the night before, then reheated in the morning.

breakfast tagine

Serves: 2
Preparation: 20 minutes
Cooking: 1¼ hours

1 tablespoon olive oil or coconut oil
1 large onion, sliced
2 garlic cloves, crushed
1 large eggplant, cubed
2 zucchini, cubed
1 small red bell pepper, seeded and thinly sliced
3¼ cups canned chopped tomatoes
1 teaspoon each ground coriander, paprika, chili powder and ground cumin
½ teaspoon cumin seeds
½ teaspoon ground cinnamon
1 teaspoon sea salt
1⅔ cups canned lima beans, rinsed and drained
1 large avocado, cut in half, pitted, peeled and cubed
2 teaspoons finely chopped mint leaves
1 small handful of parsley leaves, chopped
sea salt and freshly ground black pepper
pita bread, Chermoula Sauce (page 85) or hummus (optional), to serve

Preheat the oven to 400°F. Put the oil in a large casserole or baking dish with a lid, and add the onion, garlic, eggplant, zucchini and pepper.

Put the tomatoes in a bowl and add the coriander, paprika, chili powder, ground cumin, cumin seeds, cinnamon and salt. Mix together well, then pour this mixture over the vegetables in the casserole and stir to combine. Add the lima beans and stir gently. Cover and cook in the oven 45 minutes.

Take off the lid and check that the vegetables aren't sticking to the casserole dish. If necessary, add ¼ cup water. Season well with salt and pepper, then stir and cook another 15 to 30 minutes until the eggplant is soft. Scatter the avocado over it and sprinkle with mint and parsley, then serve with the pita bread and sauce.

Gluten-free *Soy-free* *Nut-free* *Seed-free* *Sugar-free*

Gluten-free Nut-free Seed-free

vegie head *baked beans*

Serves: 4
Preparation: 10 minutes
Cooking: 25 minutes

1 teaspoon olive oil or
  coconut oil
1 onion, cubed
1 teaspoon mustard powder
1 teaspoon tomato paste
1 teaspoon tamari soy
  sauce, regular soy sauce or
  coconut aminos
1 tablespoon brown sugar or
  coconut sugar
½ cup vegetable stock
1 cup canned chopped
  tomatoes
1⅔ cups canned lima beans
  or red kidney beans, rinsed
  and drained
sea salt and freshly ground
  black pepper
thickly sliced sourdough
  bread, fried spinach and
  mushrooms, to serve

Heat the oil in a large saucepan over high heat and fry the onion 5 to 8 minutes, stirring frequently, until softened.

Add the mustard powder, tomato paste, tamari and sugar, and stir to combine. Add the stock, tomatoes and beans. Bring to a boil over medium-high heat, then cook 10 to 15 minutes until the mixture thickens slightly and the beans are warmed through. Season with salt and pepper and serve with bread, fried spinach and mushrooms.

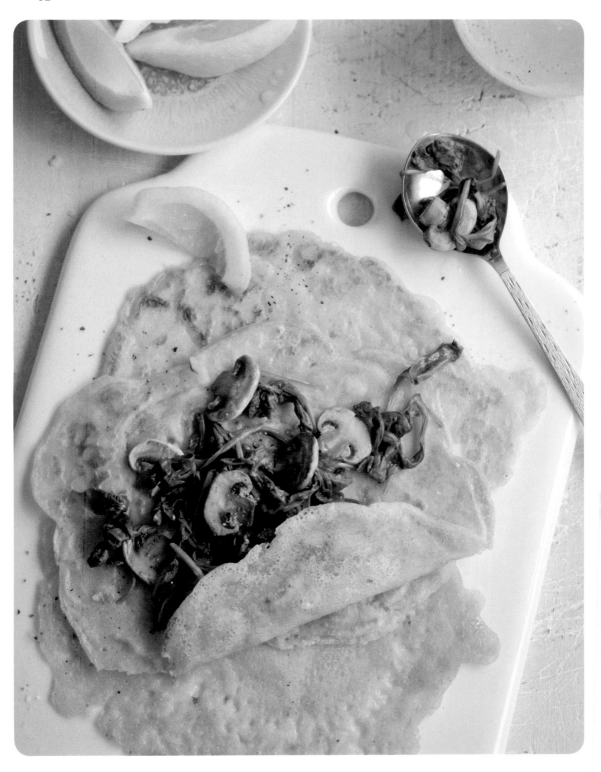

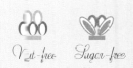

Nut-free Sugar-free

crêpes with spinach & *mushrooms*

Serves: 4
Preparation: 30 minutes,
** plus 1 hour resting**
Cooking: 30 minutes

½ cup soy milk
¼ cup vegan margarine
1 cup all-purpose flour
1 tablespoon olive oil or
  coconut oil
dairy-free yogurt and lemon
  wedges, to serve

SPINACH AND MUSHROOM
  FILLING
1 teaspoon olive oil or
  coconut oil
2¾ cups button mushrooms,
  thinly sliced
14 ounces baby spinach
1 tablespoon lemon juice
sea salt and freshly ground
  black pepper

Put the milk in a large bowl and add the margarine, flour and a pinch of salt, then add scant ¾ cup water at room temperature. Whisk, or use an electric beater, until smooth. Cover the bowl with plastic wrap, and put in the refrigerator 1 hour.

Preheat the oven to 350°F and put a heatproof plate inside to warm. To cook the crêpes, heat 1 teaspoon of the oil in a 7-inch skillet and add just enough batter to coat the bottom of the pan, tilting the pan to spread the mixture. Cook until bubbles appear on the surface, then carefully turn the crêpe over and cook the other side until lightly golden. Put the crêpe onto the warmed plate, then cover and keep warm in the oven while you cook the remaining batter.

Meanwhile, to make the filling, heat the oil in a nonstick saucepan over low heat. Add the mushrooms and fry 10 minutes, stirring frequently, or until the juices are released. Add 1 teaspoon water at a time if the mushrooms begin to stick to the pan. Add the spinach to the pan and reduce the heat to low. Cook 2 to 3 minutes until the spinach begins to wilt, then stir in the lemon juice and season with salt and pepper.

Spoon 1 tablespoon of the filling onto one edge of a crêpe. Roll it up gently. Continue with the remaining crêpes, then put the filled crêpes in an ovenproof dish and reheat in the oven 10 minutes. (Or serve them at room temperature, if you prefer.) Serve with yogurt, and a lemon wedge.

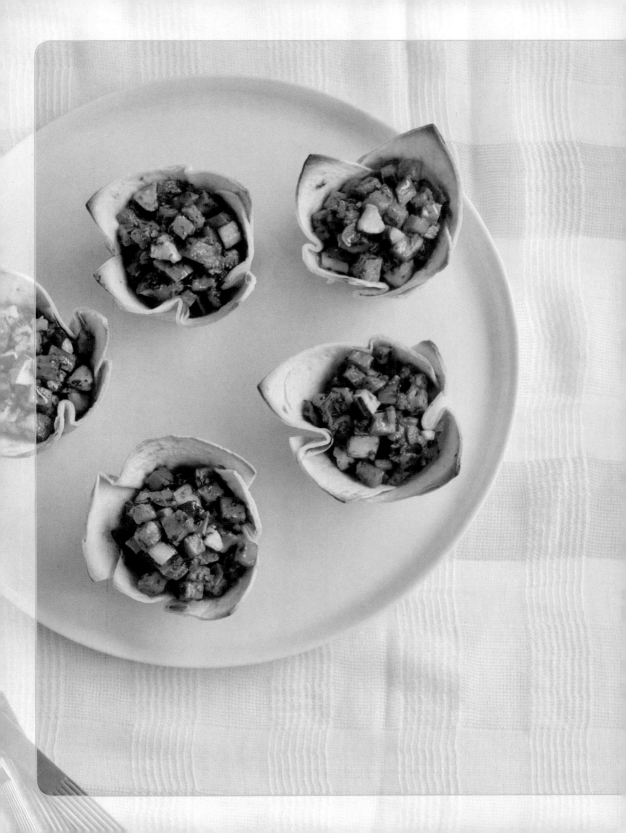

Lunches

My favorite meal of the day is definitely lunch, because it gives me my biggest burst of energy— just right for a productive afternoon. I love to eat soups at any time of the year but particularly when the weather is colder, and the Mexican Bean Soup and Moroccan Quinoa Soup are hearty dishes for any season. There are salads to suit your mood and the weather. Some are fresh and raw, such as Zucchini & Orange Carpaccio with Herbed Cheese, and others are grilled or roasted, such as Grilled Salad with Basil & Tahini Dressing or Roasted Pumpkin & Asparagus Salad. Many are suitable for making in advance and taking to work for maximum lunch envy, for picnics or when you're asked to "bring along a plate." My Sweet Potato Cups with Hummus & Walnut Pesto taste and look special and are a fun way to use tortilla wraps.

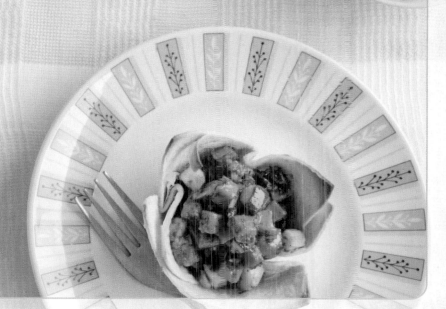

Sweet Potato Cups with
Hummus & Walnut Pesto
(page 36)

Traditional and modern Moroccan spices combine with cannellini beans and fiber- and protein-rich quinoa to make this soup a hearty meal. The soup can also be served with some crusty sourdough bread, a spoonful of hummus and a squeeze of lemon, if you like.

moroccan quinoa soup

Serves: 4–6
Preparation: 15 minutes
Cooking: 35 minutes

2 tablespoons olive oil or
   coconut oil
2 onions, finely chopped
3 garlic cloves, crushed
1 zucchini, cubed
2 cups chopped tomatoes
2 cups canned cannellini
   beans, drained and rinsed
1½ tablespoons harissa paste
1 teaspoon turmeric
1 teaspoon ground cumin
1 teaspoon ground cinnamon
¼ teaspoon sweet paprika
1 cup quinoa, rinsed and
   drained
8¾ cups vegetable stock
3 ounces kale, finely chopped
¼ cup chopped mint leaves
sea salt and freshly ground
   black pepper
dairy-free yogurt, to serve

Heat the oil in a large, heavy pot over medium heat. Add the onions and garlic, and cook 5 to 8 minutes until softened.

Add the zucchini, tomatoes, beans, harissa, spices, quinoa and stock, then season with salt and pepper and stir well. Bring to a boil over high heat, then reduce the heat to medium-high and cook 15 minutes, stirring frequently, or until the quinoa is tender and translucent.

Add the kale and cook another 5 minutes, then remove from the heat. Sprinkle the mint leaves over it and serve with a large spoonful of yogurt.

Gluten-free *Soy-free* *Nut-free* *Seed-free* *Sugar-free*

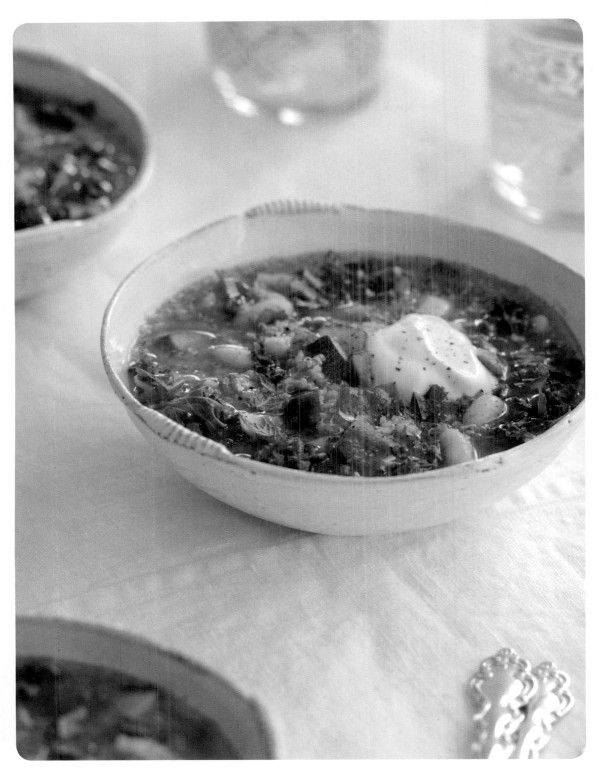

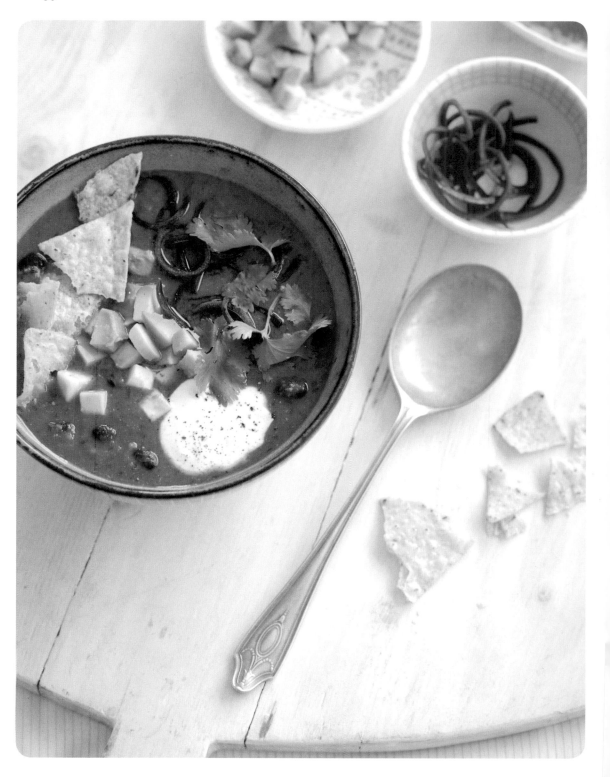

Sweet, smoky chilies and a hint of paprika give this soup the aroma and flavor that remind me of eating true Mexican food in America. I'm immediately transported to the small, wooden building with sombreros hanging on the walls, neon signs promoting cerveza (beer)—and amazing traditional food.

mexican bean soup

Serves: 6
Preparation: 20 minutes
Cooking: 40 minutes

2 tablespoons olive oil or
  coconut oil
2 onions, chopped
3 garlic cloves, crushed
12 ounces tomatoes, chopped
2 cups vegetable stock
2 cups canned red kidney
  beans, rinsed and drained
1 teaspoon smoked paprika
1 teaspoon sea salt
1 teaspoon dried oregano
1 tablespoon dried ancho
  chilies, or 1 teaspoon ancho
  or regular chili powder
1 cup canned black beans,
  rinsed and drained

TO SERVE
vegan sour cream or dairy-
  free yogurt
cubed avocado
lime wedges
crushed corn chips
finely sliced red chilies
cilantro

Heat the oil in a large, heavy pot over medium heat. Add the onions and garlic, and cook 10 minutes, or until translucent. Add the tomatoes, stock, kidney beans, paprika, salt, oregano and chilies, and return to a boil, then simmer 5 minutes.

Using a blender or food processor, blend the mixture until smooth, then add the black beans and cook another 15 minutes, or until the liquid has reduced and the black beans are thoroughly heated through. Serve with a spoonful of sour cream and top with cubed avocado, a squeeze of lime juice and a sprinkle of corn chips, red chilies and cilantro.

Gluten free

Soy free

Nut free

Seed free

Sugar free

Here is a traditional hot and sour Indian soup with herbs and spices melding together to create an authentic flavor. If you prefer your soup a little thicker, use less water or add some leftover cooked brown rice or quinoa.

rasam *soup*

Serves: 4
Preparation: 15 minutes
Cooking: 30 minutes

1 cup red lentils, rinsed and drained
scant 1⅔ cups canned chopped tomatoes
8¾ cups vegetable stock
1 teaspoon olive oil or coconut oil
1 teaspoon cumin seeds
1 teaspoon mustard seeds
8 garlic cloves, crushed
1 large onion, finely chopped
½-inch piece fresh ginger root, peeled and grated
½ teaspoon ground turmeric
½ teaspoon ground coriander
1 dried red chili or ½ teaspoon crushed chilies, or to taste
2 teaspoons tamarind paste
juice of 2 lemons
juice of 1 lime
1 large handful of cilantro, chopped

Put the lentils in a large, heavy pot and add the tomatoes and stock. Bring to a boil over high heat, then lower the heat to medium-high and cook 20 minutes, or until the lentils are soft.

Meanwhile, heat the oil in a nonstick skillet over medium heat. Add the cumin and mustard seeds to the pan, and stir-fry 30 seconds, or until the seeds begin to pop. Add the garlic and onion to the skillet and cook 10 minutes, or until the onion is translucent.

Using a blender or food processor, blend the lentil mixture until smooth. Return to low heat to keep warm.

Stir the ginger into the skillet and add the turmeric, ground coriander and dried chili, then fry 30 seconds, or until fragrant. Add the spicy onion to the blended lentils and stir in the tamarind paste, lemon juice and lime juice. Stir in the cilantro and serve.

    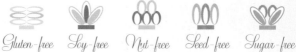

Gluten-free   Soy-free   Nut-free   Seed-free   Sugar-free

One weekend away some years ago I was treated to dinner at a fine-dining restaurant where we were served little shot glasses filled with a bright yellow soup—it was a cream of corn and lemongrass. As I sipped it, it was like a thousand fireworks going off inside my mouth. If I close my eyes, I can still remember the experience. I came home and created my own, healthier version. Serve this in bowls for lunch or in shot glasses for a flavor explosion to start a main meal.

thai corn soup

Serves: 4
Preparation: 5 minutes,
  plus making the chips
Cooking: 35 minutes

1 tablespoon olive oil or
  coconut oil
1 small leek, white part only,
  thinly sliced
1 lemongrass stalk, outer
  leaves removed, white part
  sliced
1 small red chili, seeded and
  sliced (optional)
2 cups coconut cream
2 cups fresh or frozen corn
3¼ cups vegetable stock
½ teaspoon brown sugar or
  coconut sugar
juice of 1 lime
2 kaffir lime leaves, torn
sea salt
Baked Chili Vegetable Chips
  (page 96), to serve

Heat the oil in a heavy pot over medium heat, and add the leek, lemongrass and chili. Cook 5 to 6 minutes until the leek is tender.

Add the coconut cream, corn, stock, sugar, lime juice and salt to taste, and bring to a boil. Lower the heat, and simmer 15 minutes. Using a blender or food processor, blend the ingredients until smooth and silky. Add the kaffir lime leaves and simmer another 2 minutes, then serve with the vegetable chips.

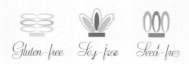

Gluten-free   Soy-free   Seed-free

Nut-free

kale & soba noodles with *ginger – chili sauce*

Serves: 4
Preparation: 15 minutes
Cooking: 20 minutes

12 ounces dried soba noodles
1 teaspoon olive oil or
  coconut oil
7 ounces smoked tofu, cubed
3 carrots, cut into matchsticks
1 large red onion, sliced
7 ounces button mushrooms,
  sliced
2 ounces red cabbage, thinly
  sliced
3 ounces kale, sliced

GINGER–CHILI SAUCE
1 garlic clove, crushed
2 tablespoons soy sauce or
  tamari soy sauce
2 tablespoons toasted sesame
  oil
¾-inch piece fresh ginger
  root, peeled and grated
juice of 1 lime
1 teaspoon chili paste
1 teaspoon brown sugar or
  coconut sugar

Put all the sauce ingredients in a small bowl and add ½ cup water. Whisk well to combine thoroughly, then set to one side to allow the flavors to develop.

Bring a large pot of water to a boil over high heat, and cook the soba noodles 4 to 5 minutes, or according to the package instructions, until soft. Drain in a colander and set to one side.

Heat the oil in a large wok or nonstick saucepan over high heat. Fry the tofu 5 minutes, turning frequently, until golden brown on all sides. Add the carrots, onion and mushrooms, and stir-fry 1 minute, or until warmed through. Add the cabbage and kale, and cook 2 minutes, or until they begin to soften. Pour the sauce mixture over the top and cook another 3 minutes, stirring frequently. Add the soba noodles and stir to combine. Cook 1 minute, or until thoroughly heated through. Remove from the heat and serve immediately.

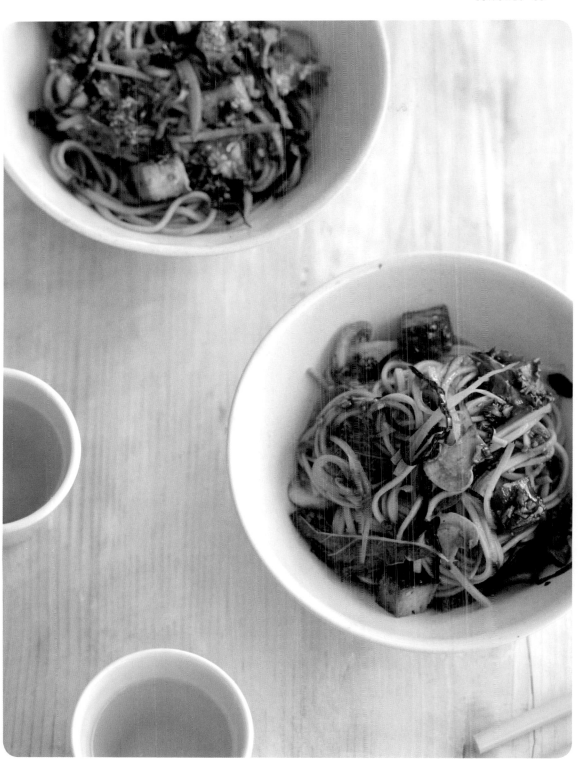

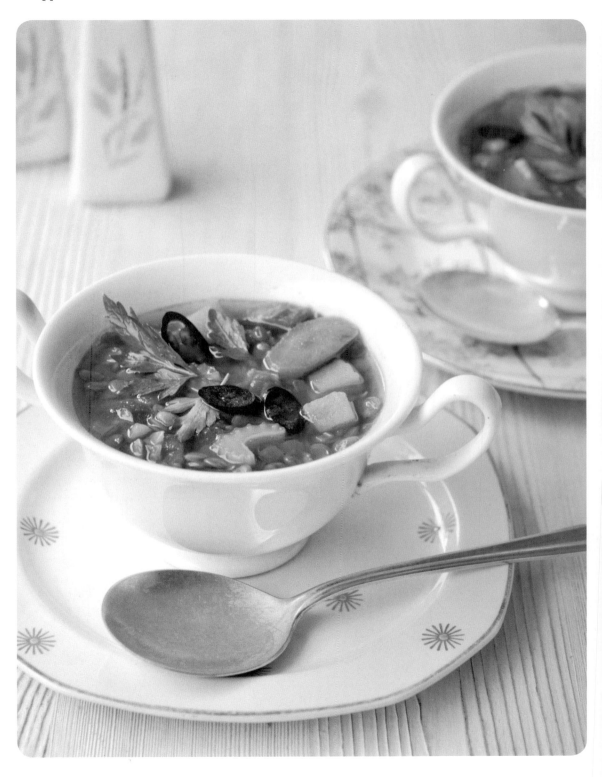

In the middle of winter, I crave this rustic soup, with its earthy flavors from the root vegetables and brown lentils and a kick from red chili. Any leftovers are perfect reheated for lunch the next day.

winter lentil soup

Serves: 6
Preparation: 15 minutes
Cooking: 55 minutes

6 ripe tomatoes
1 tablespoon olive oil or safflower oil
2 large onions, chopped
4 large garlic cloves, crushed
1 large potato, cubed
2 carrots, sliced
3 celery stalks, sliced
2¾ cups dried brown or green lentils, rinsed and drained
8¾ cups vegetable stock
1 bay leaf
1 red chili, seeded and sliced
1 handful of parsley leaves
sea salt and freshly ground black pepper

Plunge the tomatoes into boiling water for 30 seconds, then refresh in a bowl of cold water. Peel away the skins and roughly chop the flesh. Set to one side. Heat the oil in a large pot over medium heat and fry the onions 10 minutes, or until translucent. Add the garlic and cook another 2 minutes.

Add the potato, carrots and celery, and stir-fry 3 minutes, or until sizzling. Add the lentils, tomatoes, stock and the bay leaf and chili. Season well with salt and pepper. Bring to a boil over high heat, then reduce the heat to medium-high and cook 25 minutes, or until the lentils are soft. Serve sprinkled with the parsley.

Gluten-free

Soy-free

Nut-free

Seed-free

Sugar-free

My tahini dressing with a citrussy zing and the sweetness of basil lifts the flavors of grilled vegetables and makes a rich and satisfying lunch. The dressing also tastes good with falafels or as a dip.

grilled salad with basil & *tahini dressing*

Serves: 4
Preparation: 30 minutes
Cooking: 40 minutes

4 large zucchini, thinly sliced lengthwise
2 eggplants, thinly sliced lengthwise
1 fennel bulb, cut into quarters and thickly sliced
1 small head of cauliflower, thickly sliced
4 large portobello mushrooms, thinly sliced
1 tablespoon olive oil or melted coconut oil
4 large handfuls of mixed salad greens, such as dandelion, mint, parsley, cilantro, mustard, beet greens, arugula and kale, to serve

TAHINI DRESSING
¼ cup tahini
1 cup orange juice
zest and juice of ½ lemon
2 garlic cloves, crushed
¼ teaspoon ground sea salt
1 small handful of basil leaves

Preheat the oven to 200°F and put a plate inside to warm. Heat a large, ridged grill pan over medium-high heat. Put all the vegetables in a large bowl and add the oil, then toss gently to coat the vegetables and tip onto the grill pan. You may need to cook these in batches. Spread the vegetables out evenly. Cook 8 to 10 minutes, until marked with golden lines on one side. Reduce the heat, if necessary, to avoid burning.

Meanwhile, make the dressing. Put all the ingredients into a blender or food processor, then blend on high speed 30 seconds, or until the dressing is smooth and creamy. Set to one side to allow the flavors to develop.

Turn the vegetables over and cook 8 minutes, or until there are golden lines on the second side. Transfer the cooked vegetables to the warm plate while you cook the remaining batches. Put the salad greens on a large serving plate and put the cooked vegetables on top, then drizzle with the tahini dressing. Serve immediately.

Gluten-free   *Soy-free*   *Nut-free*   *Sugar-free*

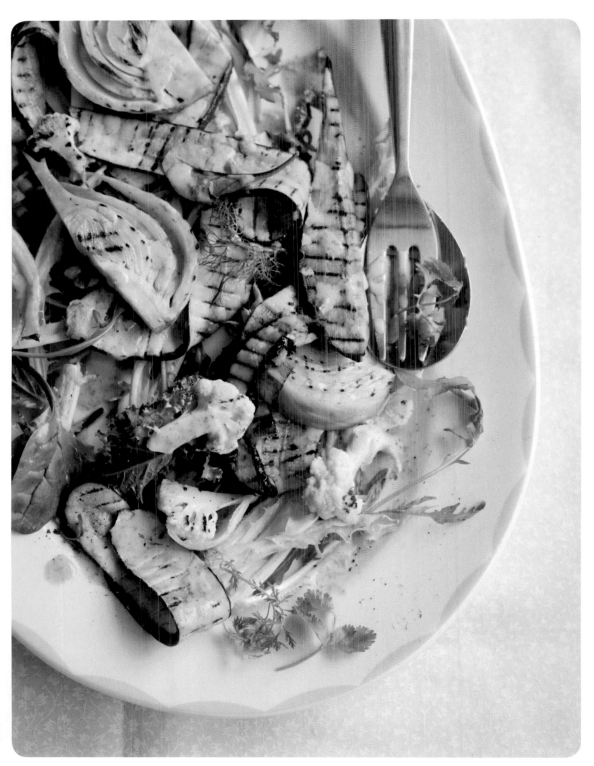

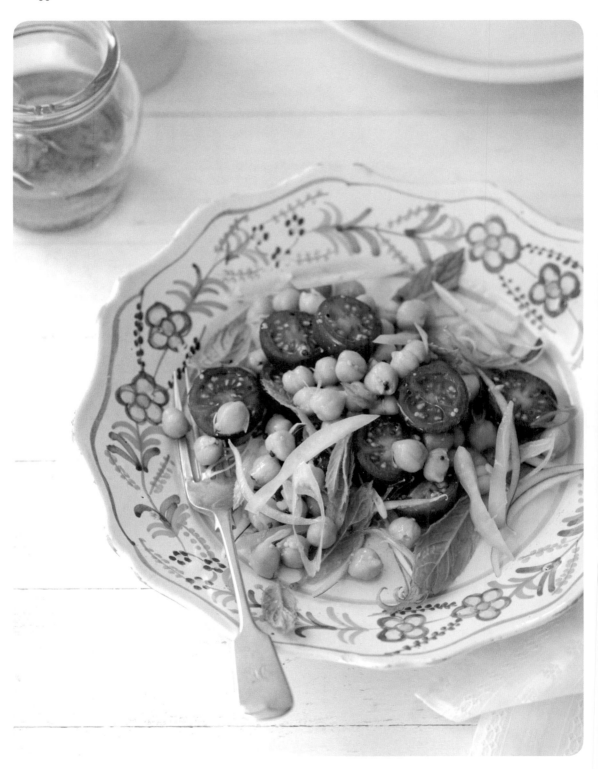

The sweetness of the tomatoes complements the nutty flavor of the chickpeas and the freshness of the mint. If you like, substitute some of the cherry tomatoes with yellow plum tomatoes to add a beautiful contrast.

chickpea, mint & tomato salad

Serves: 4
Preparation: 10 minutes

5¼–6 cups canned chickpeas, drained and rinsed
1 garlic clove, crushed
½ red onion, finely sliced
2 scallions, finely sliced
½ yellow bell pepper, seeded and thinly sliced
1 small handful of mint leaves, chopped or left whole
20 cherry tomatoes, or baby plum tomatoes, cut in half
2 tablespoons extra virgin olive oil
1 teaspoon cider vinegar
½ teaspoon wholegrain mustard
sea salt and freshly ground black pepper

Put the chickpeas in a large serving bowl and add the garlic, red onion, scallions, pepper, mint and tomatoes.

Pour the olive oil into a small bowl and add the vinegar and mustard. Whisk well, then drizzle over the salad. Season with salt and pepper, and serve immediately. Store in an airtight container in the refrigerator up to 3 days.

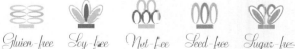

Gluten-free   Soy-free   Nut-free   Seed-free   Sugar-free

Containing fiber, protein and a large dose of antioxidants, this salad is colorful and surprisingly filling. It's perfect to take to work, on picnics, for barbecues and even for the kids' school lunches. Any beet will work well with this salad, but if you can find one of the more unusual beets, such as this pink and white salad variety, it will make the dish look particularly attractive.

sweet *super-food salad*

Serves 6
Preparation: 20 minutes

3½ cups mixed baby salad greens
2 cups cherry tomatoes, cut in half
7 ounces strawberries, sliced
2 beets, thinly sliced or grated
1 cup alfalfa sprouts
2 large cucumbers, thinly sliced
2 avocados, cut in half, peeled, pitted and sliced
1 tablespoon chia seeds
heaped 1 cup hazelnuts, roughly chopped
1 tablespoon sunflower seeds
1 tablespoon pumpkin seeds

DRESSING
1 tablespoon lemon juice
2 tablespoons cider vinegar
¼ cup extra virgin olive oil
2 teaspoons wholegrain mustard
sea salt and freshly ground black pepper

To make the dressing, put all the ingredients in a screwtop jar, cover and shake well to combine. (Alternatively, whisk in a small bowl.) Set to one side to allow the flavors to develop.

Put all the salad ingredients in a large serving bowl, and toss gently to combine. Drizzle with the dressing, then toss and serve immediately.

  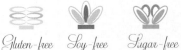

Gluten-free   Soy-free   Sugar-free   Raw

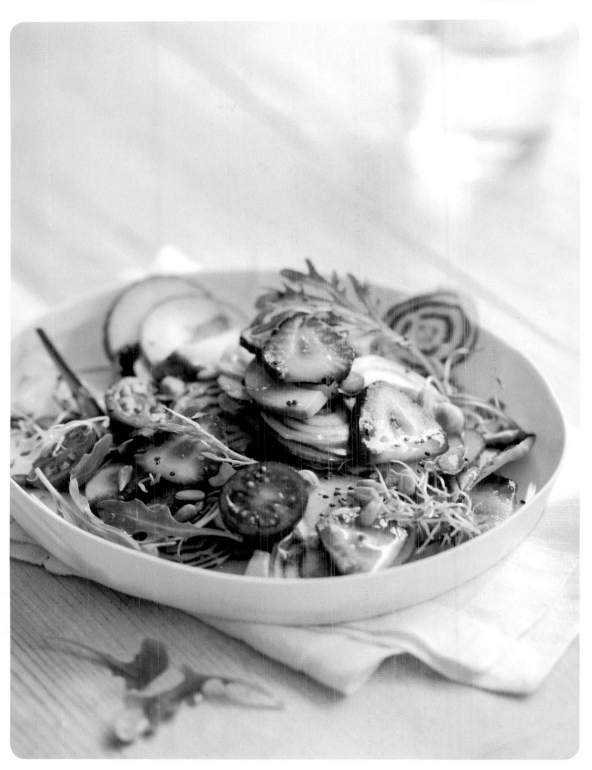

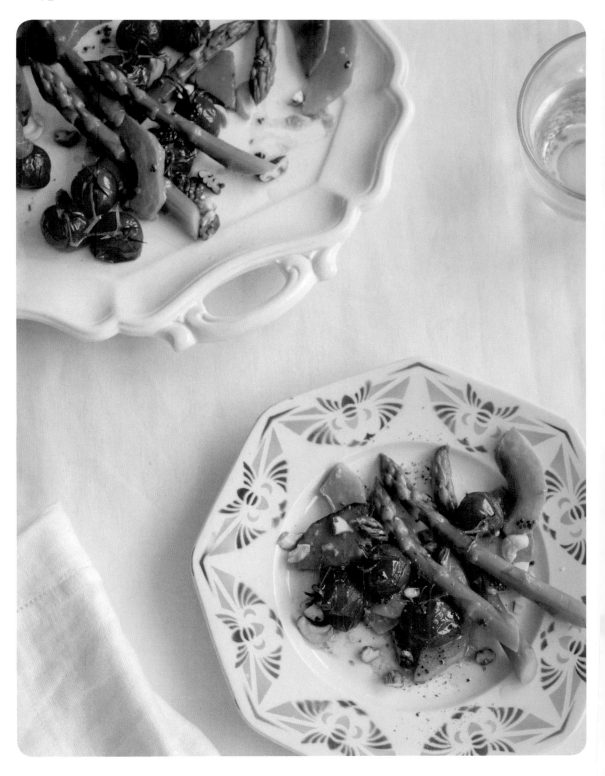

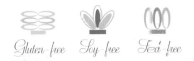

Gluten-free *Soy-free* *Egg-free*

roasted pumpkin &
asparagus salad

Serves: 4
Preparation: 15 minutes
Cooking: 25 minutes

12 asparagus spears
1¼ pounds pumpkin or
   butternut squash, peeled
   and sliced into half-moons
3 garlic cloves, crushed
2 tablespoons olive oil or
   melted coconut oil
9 ounces cherry tomatoes
1 cup mixed nuts, roughly
   chopped
sea salt and freshly ground
   black pepper

MUSTARD DRESSING
¼ cup olive oil or melted
   coconut oil
2 teaspoons brown sugar,
   brown rice syrup or agave
   syrup
1 teaspoon wholegrain
   mustard
½ teaspoon sea salt

Snap off any woody ends from the asparagus stalks at the point where they break easily, then cut the tender spears into ½-inch pieces if large, otherwise leave whole. Set to one side. Preheat the oven to 425°F.

Put the pumpkin and garlic on a baking tray and season well with salt and pepper. Add 1 tablespoon of the oil and toss to combine, then spread the mixture in the tray evenly. Roast 15 minutes. Add the cherry tomatoes and asparagus, brush with the remaining oil, then season and bake 10 minutes more, or until tender.

Meanwhile, to make the dressing, put the oil in a small bowl and add the sugar, mustard and salt, then whisk together. Remove the vegetables from the oven and set to one side to cool slightly. Toss the warm vegetables with the dressing and top with the nuts, then serve.

The sweet orange and the herby saltiness of the cheese are matched perfectly with the zucchini in this simple and fresh-tasting dish. You could also add some grated beet or fried tempeh to make it more substantial.

zucchini & orange carpaccio
with herbed cheese

Serves: 4
Preparation: 15 minutes,
  plus making the cheese

2 oranges
2 tablespoons good-quality
  extra virgin olive oil
1 tablespoon lemon juice
1 pound zucchini, preferably
  a mixture of green and
  yellow, thinly sliced
¼ quantity Herbed Almond
  Cheese (page 22), crumbled
¼ cup mint leaves, finely
  sliced or left whole
¼ cup basil leaves, finely
  sliced or left whole
sea salt and freshly ground
  black pepper

Using a sharp knife, cut a thin slice of peel and pith from each end of an orange. Put the orange, cut-side down, on a plate and cut off the peel and pith in strips. Remove any remaining pith. Cut out each segment, leaving the membrane behind. Set to one side. Squeeze the remaining juice from the membrane into a small bowl. Repeat with the second orange.

Pour the olive oil into the bowl with the orange juice and add the lemon juice and a pinch of salt. Arrange the zucchini slices and orange segments on a serving plate, overlapping them slightly. Add the herbed cheese and sprinkle with the herbs. Drizzle with the dressing, grind some pepper over it and serve.

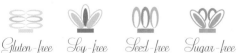

Gluten-free Soy-free Seed-free Sugar-free Raw

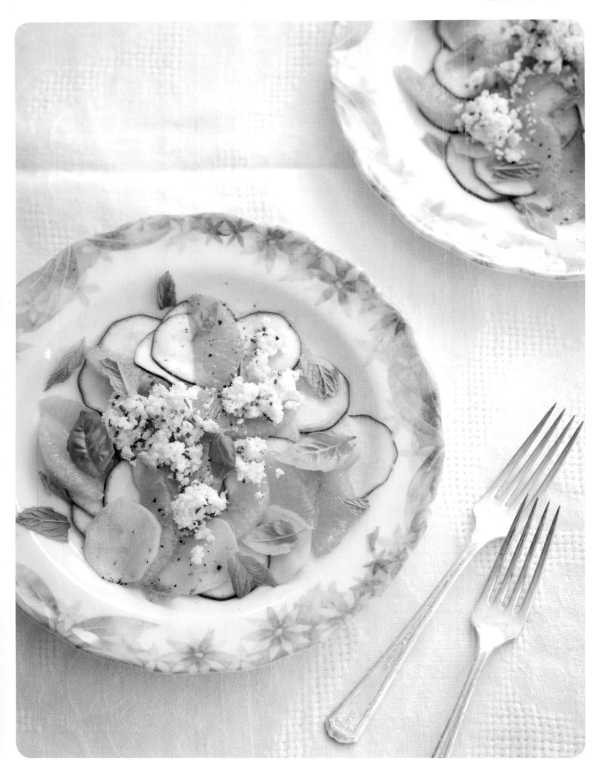

I made this salad for one of my clients who has to follow a very limited diet. It just goes to show that even the most simple of ingredients can be turned into something enticing. The salad can be served warm, as here, or cold.

noodle, zucchini &
avocado salad

Serves: 4
Preparation: 15 minutes
Cooking: 5 minutes

12 ounces brown rice noodles
2 zucchini, thinly sliced
1 tablespoon black sesame
  seeds, and mixed baby
  salad greens, to serve

AVOCADO DRESSING
2 avocados, cut in half,
  peeled and pitted
1 cup coconut milk
2 handfuls of basil leaves
1 teaspoon sea salt
2 tablespoons toasted
  sesame oil
2 teaspoons mirin or
  rice wine
2 teaspoons white wine
  vinegar

Bring a large pot of water to a boil over high heat. Add the rice noodles and zucchini slices, then reduce the heat to medium and cook 2 minutes. Drain in a colander and rinse under cold water, then set to one side to cool.

To make the dressing, put the avocados into a blender or food processor and add the coconut milk, basil, salt, oil, mirin and vinegar. Blend until smooth.

Tip the drained noodles and zucchini back into the pan and add the dressing. Toss until coated in the dressing. Sprinkle with sesame seeds and serve immediately with the salad greens.

Gluten-free

Soy-free

Sugar-free

curried chickpea patties with satay dipping sauce

Serves: 4
Preparation: 20 minutes
Cooking: 1 hour, plus cooling

⅓ cup brown rice
3 cups canned chickpeas, rinsed and drained
scant ½ cup coconut milk
½ teaspoon brown sugar or coconut sugar
⅔ cup fresh breadcrumbs
1 teaspoon mild curry powder
½ teaspoon cumin seeds
½ teaspoon onion powder
1 teaspoon sea salt
2 tablespoons olive oil or coconut oil
green salad, to serve

SATAY DIPPING SAUCE
1 cup unsalted dry-roasted peanuts
⅓ cup coconut milk
1 garlic clove
½ teaspoon soy sauce, tamari soy sauce or coconut aminos
1 tablespoon toasted sesame oil
2 teaspoons brown sugar or coconut sugar
½ teaspoon tamarind paste
2 teaspoons crushed chilies

Bring a large pot of water to a boil over high heat. Add the rice and cook 35 to 40 minutes, or according to the package instructions, until tender. Drain in a colander and set to one side to cool.

Meanwhile, to make the satay sauce, put the peanuts into a food processor and blend into a fine paste, then add the remaining sauce ingredients and ⅓ cup water. Blend until smooth and combined, then set to one side.

Put the chickpeas into a blender or food processor and pulse until chopped. Add the coconut milk, sugar, breadcrumbs, curry powder, cumin seeds, onion powder, salt and rice, then blend to combine. Heat 1 tablespoon of the oil in a nonstick skillet over medium heat.

Using a spoon, scoop out golf-ball-sized pieces of mixture and form into little patties. Fry in the oil 3 to 4 minutes until golden on one side. You will probably have to do this in batches. Turn the patties over and cook 2 minutes on the other side. Remove from the pan and keep warm. Continue until all the mixture is cooked, adding more oil as necessary. Serve with the dipping sauce and green salad.

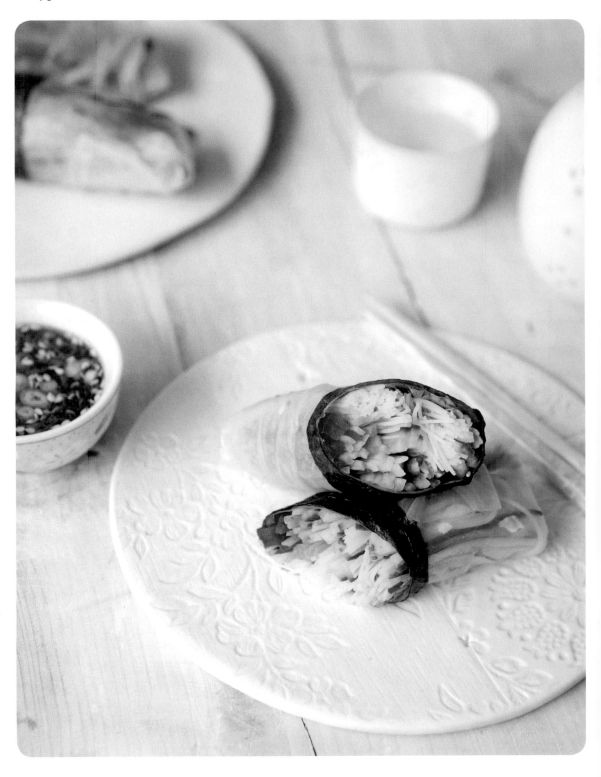

The trick to making easy rolls is to have everything cut up and ready to assemble, then it takes moments to complete.

rice paper & nori rolls

Serves: 4
Preparation: 25 minutes,
plus 2 minutes soaking

1¾ ounces rice noodles
8 rice paper sheets
2 carrots, cut into
 matchsticks
1 cucumber, cut into
 matchsticks
½ red bell pepper, seeded
 and cut into matchsticks
½ cup almonds, finely
 chopped
1 tablespoon chia seeds
1 handful of mint leaves,
 finely chopped
1 handful of cilantro, finely
 chopped
2 nori sheets, cut into
 quarters

SESAME DIPPING SAUCE
¼ cup tamari soy sauce or
 coconut aminos
½ scallion, finely sliced
1 teaspoon mirin or rice wine
 vinegar
2 teaspoons toasted sesame
 oil
1 teaspoon brown sugar or
 coconut sugar
1 teaspoon crushed chilies
1 teaspoon sesame seeds

To make the sauce, put all the ingredients in a bowl and whisk together. Set aside to allow the flavors to develop.

Put the rice noodles in a saucepan and pour boiling water over them to cover generously. Let soak 2 minutes, then drain thoroughly in a colander.

Pour boiling water into a large heatproof bowl or saucepan to a depth of ½ inch. Take a rice paper sheet and submerge it 10 to 15 seconds until it becomes transparent and flimsy. Carefully lift it out and lay it flat on a plate, then fill it as follows.

Starting close to the edge of the rice paper nearest to you, start to make a narrow layer of filling along that horizontal edge, using a one-eighth portion of rice noodles. Now layer a one-eighth portion each of carrot, cucumber pepper, almonds, chia seeds, mint and cilantro on top. Pick up the lower edge of the rice paper and tuck it over the filling, then, using flat hands, make one rolling movement to cover the filling in some of the rice paper. Tuck in the sides and roll again tightly to finish.

Put the rice paper roll on one quarter of a nori sheet and roll it up in the nori sheet. Set to one side and repeat with the remaining rice paper sheets. Cut each roll in half and serve with the dipping sauce.

Gluten-free

Nut-free

tempura pumpkin stacks with ginger dressing

Serves: 4
Preparation: 30 minutes
Cooking: 25 minutes

safflower oil or sunflower oil, for deep-frying
1¾ cups all-purpose flour
½ cup cornstarch
1 teaspoon baking powder
a pinch of sea salt
¼ teaspoon mustard powder
2 teaspoons white sesame seeds
2 teaspoons black sesame seeds
2¼ pounds pumpkin or butternut squash, peeled, seeded, and sliced into half-circles ⅛-inch thick
7 ounces salad greens
Tamari Spiced Nuts & Seeds (page 94), to serve (optional)

GINGER DRESSING
1 teaspoon sesame oil
½-inch piece fresh ginger root, peeled and grated
1 tablespoon soy sauce or tamari soy sauce
1 teaspoon brown rice syrup, agave syrup or brown sugar
juice of ½ lemon
juice of 1 lime
1 scallion, white part only, finely sliced

Preheat the oven to 200°F. Put a wire rack on a baking sheet and put inside the oven to warm. Put all the ingredients for the dressing in a screwtop jar, cover and shake well to combine. (Alternatively, whisk in a small bowl.) Set to one side to allow the flavors to develop.

Heat a wok, a large pot or a deep-fryer with the oil for deep-frying to 340°F (test by frying a small cube of bread—it should brown in 40 seconds). Sift 1 cup of the flour with the cornstarch, baking powder, salt and mustard into a large bowl. Slowly pour in 2 cups water and whisk together until smooth. The mixture should be the consistency of heavy cream.

Put all the sesame seeds in a nonstick skillet and dry-fry over low heat 30 seconds, shaking the pan constantly, until just beginning to brown. Remove from the heat and set aside.

Dust each pumpkin piece with the remaining flour, and then dip it into the batter to coat well, dipping a few times if necessary. Put some pumpkin pieces into the hot oil and let fry 4 minutes or until lightly golden. Lift out with a slotted spoon. Arrange on the wire rack and put into the oven while you fry the remaining pumpkin. Layer the pumpkin slices over the salad greens and sprinkle with the sesame seeds and spiced nuts and seeds, if you like. Serve drizzled with the dressing.

Nut-free

chinese scallion pancakes with *dipping sauce*

Serves: 4
Preparation: 20 minutes,
 plus 30 minutes resting
Cooking: 15 minutes

¼-ounce envelope
 (2¾ teaspoons) fast-action
 dry yeast
a pinch of sugar
1 cup all-purpose flour, plus
 extra for dusting
½ cup wholewheat flour
3 tablespoons safflower oil or
 sunflower oil, plus extra
 for greasing
2 tablespoons toasted
 sesame oil
4 scallions, finely chopped

GINGER DIPPING SAUCE
3 tablespoons soy sauce or
 tamari soy sauce
1 tablespoon white wine
 vinegar
1 teaspoon mirin
1 teaspoon chili oil
2 teaspoons toasted
 sesame oil
½ teaspoon brown sugar or
 coconut sugar, or brown
 rice syrup or agave syrup
1 garlic clove, crushed
¼-inch piece fresh ginger
 root, peeled and grated
1 scallion, thinly sliced

To make the dipping sauce, put all the ingredients in a small serving bowl and whisk together. Set to one side for the flavors to develop. Put the yeast in a small bowl, and add ½ cup warm water and the sugar, then whisk together. Sift the flours into a large bowl, and tip in any bran remaining in the sifter. Stir in the yeast mixture, then use your hands to incorporate all the flour into the liquid. (Alternatively, sift the flours into a food processor. With the blades turning, slowly pour in the yeast mixture, until the mixture forms a dough.)

Turn the dough onto a lightly floured surface and knead 2 to 4 minutes until smooth (Or, if your machine has a kneading function, set this for 1 minute.) Lightly oil a large bowl, add the dough and cover with a damp dish towel. Leave in a warm place 30 minutes.

Divide the dough into 20 pieces, roll them into balls, then put them on a floured surface and roll them flat. Brush some sesame oil over each one, and sprinkle with the scallions. Roll the dough circles into a cigar shape, then roll them up again from one end to the other, to make a spiral. With the spiral laying flat, roll the dough into a thin circle. Heat the safflower oil in a large skillet and fry the pancakes 2 to 3 minutes on each side. Serve with the dipping sauce.

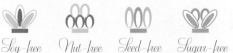

Soy-free   Nut-free   Seed-free   Sugar-free

lemon, artichoke & baby spinach spaghetti

Serves: 4
Preparation: 10 minutes
Cooking: 15 minutes

12 ounces wholewheat
   spaghetti
6 ounces bottled or canned
   marinated artichoke hearts,
   drained and cut into
   quarters
juice of 2 lemons
2 teaspoons finely grated
   lemon zest
2 large handfuls of basil
   leaves
1 cup baby spinach leaves
extra virgin olive oil, for
   drizzling
sea salt and freshly ground
   black pepper

Bring a large pot of salted water to a boil over high heat, add
the spaghetti and cook 10 to 12 minutes, or according to the
package instructions, until just tender. Drain the spaghetti in a
colander, reserving ¼ cup of the cooking liquid, and return both
the pasta and the reserved water to the pan.

Add the artichoke hearts, lemon juice and zest, basil and spinach
to the pan and mix well.

Drizzle the olive oil over the pasta to taste and serve with plenty
of black pepper.

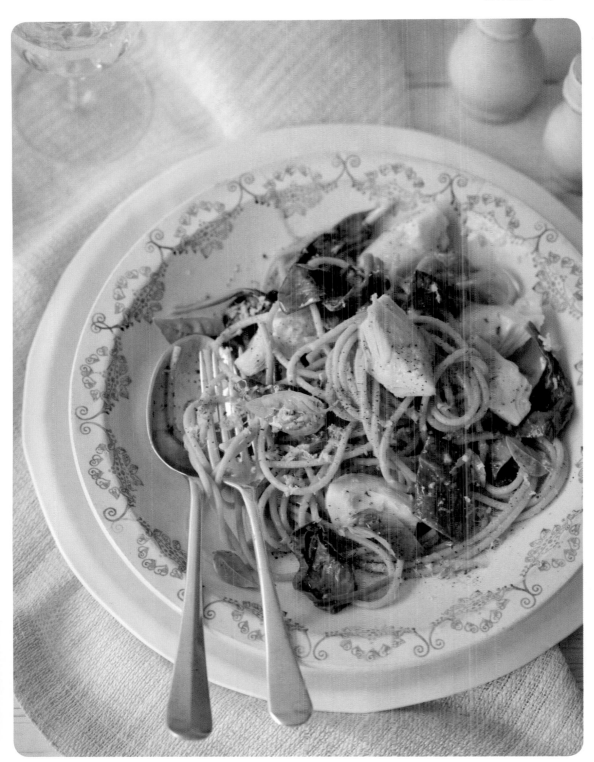

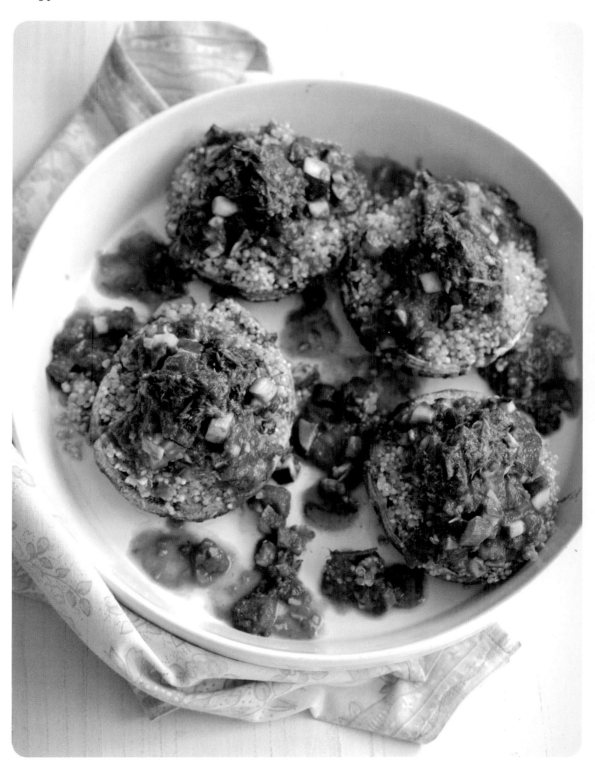

moroccan stuffed mushrooms

Serves: 4
Preparation: 20 minutes
Cooking: 45 minutes

1 heaped cup quinoa, rinsed
  and drained
2 teaspoons tamari soy
  sauce or soy sauce, or to
  taste
8 large portobello
  mushrooms, stems removed
  and finely chopped, and
  caps set aside
4 cups canned chopped
  tomatoes
4 garlic cloves, crushed
8 ounces zucchini, finely
  chopped
1 teaspoon chermoula paste
  or chili powder, or to taste
¼ cup chopped basil leaves
2 teaspoons sweet paprika
1 teaspoon ground turmeric
½ teaspoon ground
  cinnamon
sea salt and freshly ground
  black pepper
salad greens, to serve

CHERMOULA SAUCE
1 large handful of cilantro
2 large handfuls of parsley
  leaves
4 garlic cloves
½ teaspoon sea salt
2 teaspoons ground cumin
1 teaspoon sweet paprika
¼ teaspoon crushed chilies
2 saffron threads
⅓ cup extra virgin olive oil
juice of 1 large lemon

Preheat the oven to 350°F, and line a baking tray with baking parchment. Put the quinoa in a pan and add 1 ¼ cups water. Bring to a boil over high heat, then reduce the heat to medium-low and simmer 15 minutes, or until tender and translucent, and the water has mostly been absorbed. Drain in a strainer, then tip back into the pan. Season to taste with pepper and tamari.

Meanwhile, put the mushroom caps on the prepared baking tray, then set aside.

Put the tomatoes in a saucepan over medium heat and add the garlic, zucchini, chermoula paste, chopped mushroom stems, basil, paprika, turmeric and cinnamon. Bring to a boil and then reduce the heat to a simmer. Season with salt and pepper. Cook 10 minutes, stirring frequently, then remove from the heat.

Meanwhile, put all the chermoula sauce ingredients into a blender or food processor and blend until smooth.

Spoon an eighth of the quinoa into each mushroom, and top with the tomato mixture. Cook the mushrooms in the oven 15 minutes and serve with the salad greens and a spoonful of the chermoula sauce

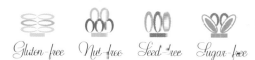

Gluten-free   Nut-free   Seed-free   Sugar-free

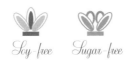

Soy-free   Sugar-free

sweet potato cups with hummus & walnut pesto

Serves: 3–6
Preparation: 30 minutes,
  plus cooling and making
  the hummus
Cooking: 1 hour

9 ounces sweet potato, cut
  into small cubes
1 tablespoon olive oil or
  coconut oil, plus extra for
  greasing
½ zucchini, finely chopped
3 flour tortillas
1 large handful of basil leaves
1 small handful of parsley
  leaves
2 cups baby spinach leaves
¼ cup walnuts
¼ cup good-quality extra
  virgin olive oil
1 garlic clove, crushed
a squeeze of lemon juice, or
  to taste
sea salt and freshly ground
  black pepper
1 cup hummus, such as
  Roasted Garlic & Hazelnut
  Hummus (page 98)

Preheat the oven to 400°F. Put the sweet potato in a bowl and add the oil. Mix well to coat thoroughly and tip onto a baking tray. Roast 30 minutes, then add the zucchini to the tray. Roast 15 minutes more, or until tender.

While the vegetables are cooking, cut each tortilla into quarters and, using a small amount of oil, grease six muffin cups. Press 1 piece of tortilla inside a muffin cup and smooth into the edges to line the cup, then add a second piece at an angle and smooth in the same way. Leave the edges overhanging, to create a tortilla "cup." Set aside.

Put the basil into a blender or food processor and add the parsley and spinach leaves, then blend until they are well combined. Add the walnuts, olive oil, garlic and lemon juice. Season with salt and pepper, and blend into a smooth paste to make a pesto.

When the sweet potato is cooked, set the baking tray aside to cool. When the vegetables are cool, tip them into a large mixing bowl, and combine with 2 tablespoons of walnut pesto. Spoon the sweet potato and zucchini mixture into each tortilla cup and bake 15 minutes, or until the tortillas are golden brown. Top with a large spoonful of hummus and serve with the remaining pesto. The pesto can be stored in a sterilized jar in the refrigerator up to 1 week or frozen up to 1 month.

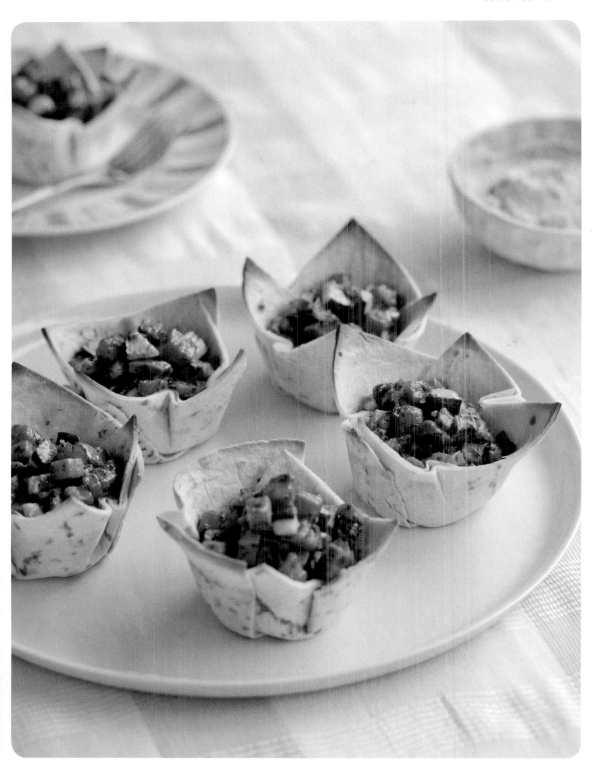

This simple curry can be changed in many ways to suit what you have in your cupboard or for a different flavor emphasis. You can add potatoes, red kidney beans, spinach, kale or pumpkin or you can increase the chili and garam masala, or try some lime juice and a dash of coconut cream.

super-fast chickpea curry

Serves: 4
Preparation: 15 minutes,
  plus making the parathas
Cooking: 30 minutes

1 tablespoon olive oil or
  coconut oil
2 onions, finely chopped
3 garlic cloves, crushed
¼-inch piece fresh ginger
  root, peeled and grated
1 teaspoon yellow mustard
  seeds
1 teaspoon cumin seeds
1½ teaspoons garam masala
1 teaspoon ground turmeric
1 teaspoon ground cumin
2 teaspoons dried fenugreek
  leaves or 1 teaspoon dried
  fenugreek
2 cups canned chopped
  tomatoes
1 large tomato, chopped
6 cups canned chickpeas,
  rinsed and drained
1 teaspoon crushed chilies, or
  to taste (optional)
2 tablespoons chopped
  cilantro
sea salt
Garlic Parathas (page 27),
  to serve

Heat the oil in a large, heavy pot over medium heat. Add the onions, garlic and ginger, and cook 5 to 8 minutes until softened. Add 1 teaspoon of water if the onions start to stick on the bottom of the pot.

Move the cooked onions to one side of the pot, and add the mustard seeds and cumin seeds to the other side. Leave them a few seconds, then start to move them with a spoon and stir-fry 30 seconds, or until they begin to pop. Stir them into the onions and add 2 teaspoons water. Add the garam masala, turmeric, ground cumin and fenugreek, and stir well. The mixture will become a thick, brown paste.

Add the canned and fresh tomatoes, the chickpeas and 2 cups water. Stir well and bring to a boil, then reduce the heat and simmer over medium-high heat 15 minutes. Season with salt and add the crushed chilies, if using. Scatter the cilantro over it and serve with the parathas

Gluten-free   *Soy-free*   *Nut-free*   *Seed-free*   *Sugar-free*

Sugar-free

creamy bean *quesadillas*

Serves: 4
Preparation: 15 minutes,
  plus making the sauce
Cooking: 10 minutes

2 cups canned red kidney
  beans, rinsed and drained
1 teaspoon ground cumin
¼ teaspoon ground
  cinnamon
3 tablespoons tahini
1 teaspoon paprika
1 teaspoon crushed chilies
3 garlic cloves
1 avocado
8 wholewheat or white flour
  tortillas
1 quantity Vegan Cheese
  Sauce (page 23)
½ cup mild salsa, plus extra
  to serve
1 large handful of cilantro
2 ounces red cabbage, very
  thinly sliced
1 small handful of baby
  spinach leaves, torn
1 red onion, very thinly sliced

Put the kidney beans into a food processor and add the cumin, cinnamon, tahini, paprika, crushed chilies and garlic. Blend until smooth.

Cut the avocado in half, remove the pit and peel, then cut into chunks and put into a small bowl. Roughly mash with a fork.

Heat a large, nonstick skillet over medium heat. Lay 4 tortillas on the work surface. Spread a layer of the spicy kidney bean mixture over each tortilla, then add a large spoonful of the vegan cheese sauce.

Spoon the avocado over the tortillas and top with some salsa, cilantro, red cabbage, spinach and slices of red onion. Put a tortilla on top of each to make quesadillas. Put 1 quesadilla into the skillet. Dry-fry on each side 1 minute, or until golden brown. Repeat with the remaining quesadillas. Serve with the remaining sauce and the salsa.

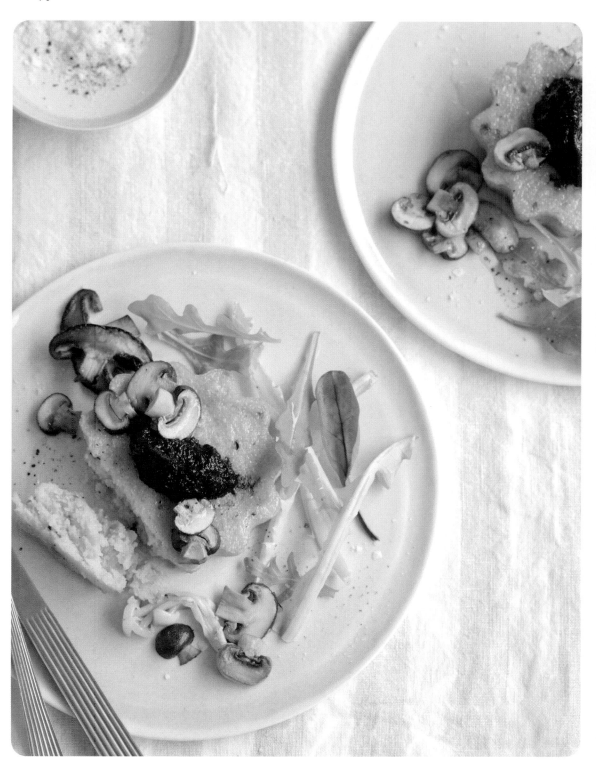

Gluten-free *Nut-free* *Sugar-free*

mushroom & roasted
beet *polenta nests*

Serves: 6
Preparation: 20 minutes,
   plus 1 hour chilling
Cooking: 1½ hours,
   plus cooling

2 tablespoons olive oil, plus
   extra for greasing
2⅔ cups boiling vegetable
   stock, or liquid called for
   in the polenta package
   instructions
1½ cups fine polenta
2 teaspoons crushed chilies
2 large beets, cut into
   quarters
1 garlic clove
2 tablespoons lemon juice
1 teaspoon ground cumin
1 tablespoon vegan cream
   cheese
1 teaspoon safflower oil or
   sunflower oil
1 pound, 5 ounces mixed
   mushrooms, such as
   button, chestnut, shiitake
   and enoki, sliced
sea salt and freshly ground
   black pepper
green salad, to serve

Preheat the oven to 350°F and lightly grease six nonstick
individual tart pans. Pour the boiling stock into a medium
saucepan, return to the boil and add 1 teaspoon salt. Pour in
the polenta in a fine stream, whisking as you pour.

Add the olive oil and crushed chilies, and season with pepper,
then whisk until combined. Cook 5 minutes, or according to
the package instructions, then pour into the prepared tart pans.
Cool, then chill in the refrigerator 1 hour, or until firm.

Meanwhile, wrap the quartered beets in foil, and bake
1 hour. Unwrap and let cool. Put the beets in a blender or
food processor and add the garlic, lemon juice, cumin and
cream cheese. Blend together until smooth. Season with
salt and pepper, then set aside.

Bake the polenta tarts 30 minutes, or until cooked and crisp.
Meanwhile, heat the safflower oil in a large skillet over medium-
high heat and add the mushrooms. Fry 10 minutes, or until
golden. Season lightly with salt and pepper and remove from
the heat. Carefully remove the cooked polenta from the
tart pans and put a spoonful of the beet spread on top. Put
the mushrooms on the spread and serve with the green salad.

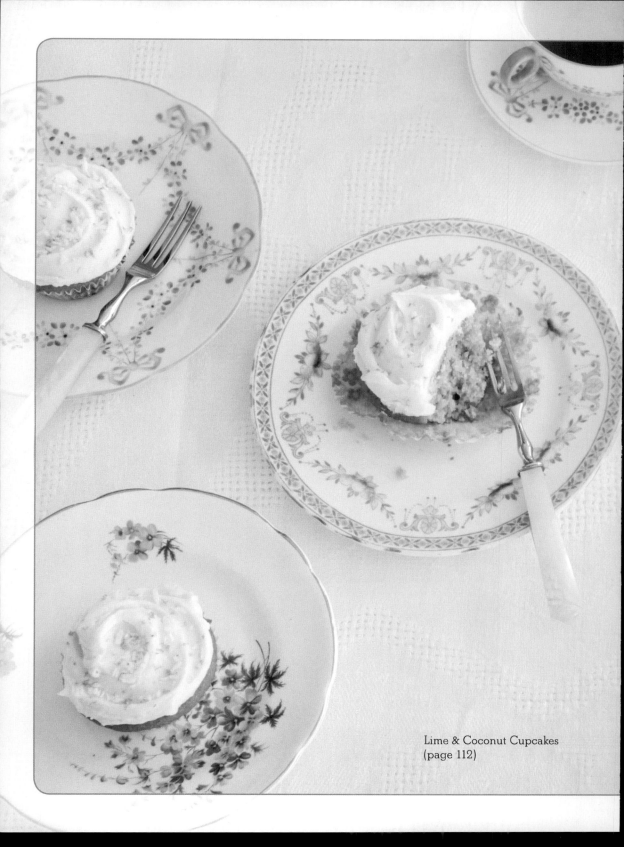

Lime & Coconut Cupcakes
(page 112)

Snacks & Treats

Pop some healthy treats into your handbag or lunchbox to stave away the 3pm craving monster, which can lead the cleanest of diets into a tailspin of sugar and unhealthy fats. Whether for midmorning or midafternoon, these snacks and treats are sure to appeal to the fussy little ones in your family (or even the bigger ones), and they also make great party treats. Seasoned treats include Tamari Spiced Nuts & Seeds (great to sprinkle over salads as well), Roasted Garlic & Hazelnut Hummus, plus Baked Chili Vegetable Chips or Savory Cookies to go with a drink. Keep your energy up with a bit of fruity sweetness from Cherry Coconut Crunch Bars or Spiced Apple Tea Cake, and cool the kids down during a hot afternoon with my Peach, Orange Blossom & Coconut Popsicles.

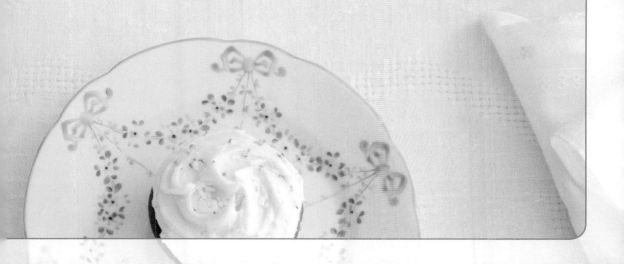

Nutritious nuts and seeds, coated in a lightly spiced, salty sauce, make a perfect party nibble or snack to eat on the run. I keep a small jar of them in my purse in case of a hunger emergency. They can also be sprinkled over salads.

tamari spiced nuts & *seeds*

Serves: 4
Preparation: 10 minutes
Cooking: 20 minutes,
 plus cooling

1 cup almonds
½ cup walnuts
¼ cup soy nuts or dried
 edamame
¼ cup pecans
½ cup pumpkin seeds
1 cup sunflower seeds
¼ cup sesame seeds
¼ cup tamari soy sauce or
 soy sauce, or to taste
1 teaspoon toasted sesame oil
½ teaspoon brown sugar or
 coconut sugar
½ teaspoon ground
 cinnamon
½ teaspoon ground allspice

Preheat the oven to 350°F and line a baking tray with baking parchment. Put all the nuts and seeds in a large bowl and toss to mix well.

Put the tamari in a small bowl and add the sesame oil, sugar and spices, then whisk together. Pour this mixture over the nuts and stir to combine until the nuts are thoroughly coated.

Arrange the nuts everly over the prepared baking tray and bake 10 minutes, then shake the baking tray to toss the nuts and return it to the oven to cook 10 minutes more. Let cool, then serve. Store in an airtight container up to 4 weeks.

Gluten-free

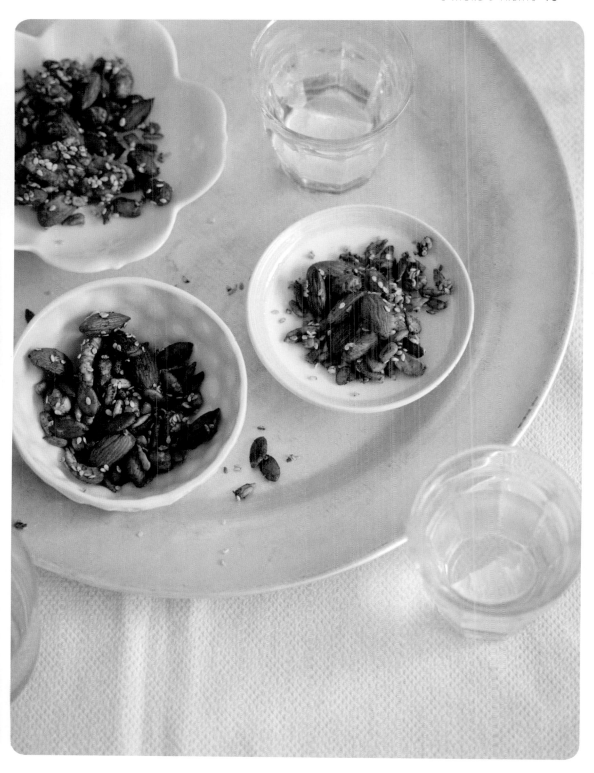

I love making a huge bowl of these healthy chips, which can be prepared with other vegetables as well. I often make them using carrot, daikon radish or pumpkin. It's a great way to use up any root or starchy vegetables you have in your vegetable rack.

baked chili vegetable chips

Serves: 2
Preparation: 20 minutes
Cooking: 35 minutes

2 beets
1 sweet potato
1 parsnip
1 potato
2 tablespoons olive oil or
  melted coconut oil
½ teaspoon sea salt
½ teaspoon garlic powder
½ teaspoon dried basil
½ teaspoon dried oregano
½ teaspoon dried rosemary
2 teaspoons crushed chilies
1 teaspoon paprika

Preheat the oven to 350°F. Use a wire rack on a baking tray to cook the chips—this will ensure they are evenly cooked and crisp up well.

Slice all the vegetables into uniformly thin slices, preferably using a mandoline. Put the vegetables in a large bowl and drizzle with the oil. Sprinkle the flavorings over them and mix well to cover the slices completely. Arrange the slices on the rack in a single layer and bake 10 to 12 minutes, until crisp and lightly golden. You may have to do this in batches. Let cool and serve. Store in an airtight container up to 3 days.

Gluten-free   Soy-free   Nut-free   Seed-free   Sugar-free

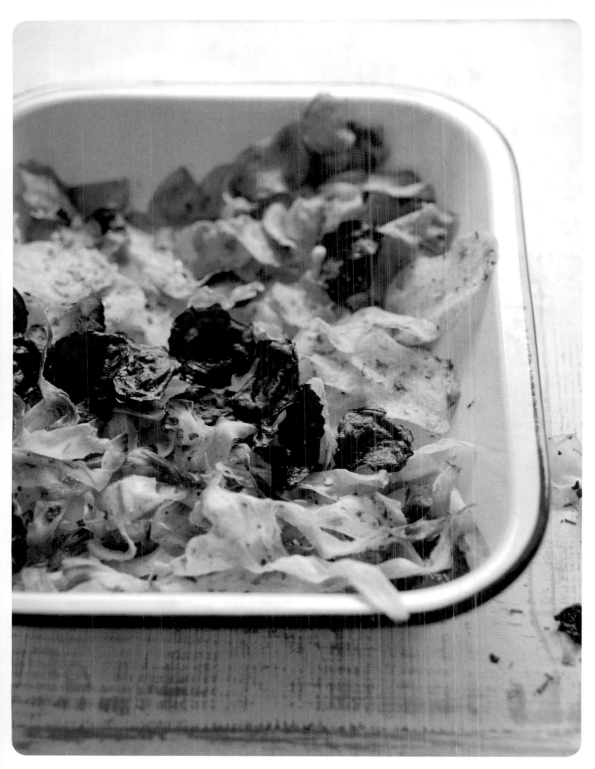

The Spanish make a picada sauce using hazelnuts, tomato, garlic, bread and oil, and this was the inspiration for my nutty hummus.

roasted garlic & hazelnut hummus

Serves: 2
Preparation: 15 minutes
Cooking: 30 minutes,
  plus cooling

3 garlic cloves, unpeeled
½ cup hazelnuts
3 cups canned chickpeas,
  rinsed and drained
3 tablespoons good-quality
  extra virgin olive oil, plus
  extra to serve
2 tablespoons vegetable stock
juice of 1 large lemon
1 teaspoon sea salt
¼ teaspoon sweet paprika
pita bread and vegetable
  sticks, to serve

Preheat the oven to 400°F and line a baking tray with baking parchment. Put the garlic on the prepared baking tray and roast 15 minutes. Add the hazelnuts to the tray and roast another 15 minutes.

Set the hazelnuts and garlic to one side until cool to the touch. Using a clean dish towel, take a handful of hazelnuts and rub off the skins. Repeat with the remaining hazelnuts. Put the nuts in a food processor and squeeze in the roasted garlic from its skin. Blend 2 minutes, or until the hazelnuts have released their oil.

Add the chickpeas and blend 30 seconds, then slowly drizzle in the oil with the blades still turning. Add the stock, lemon juice, salt and paprika, and blend until smooth. Serve drizzled with extra olive oil, with pita bread and vegetable sticks.

Gluten-free

Soy-free

Seed-free

Sugar-free

roasted afghani *chickpeas*

Serves: 4
Preparation: 5 minutes
Cooking: 40 minutes

1 tablespoon olive oil or
   melted coconut oil
zest and juice of 1 lemon
1 teaspoon paprika
½ teaspoon turmeric
3 cups canned chickpeas,
   rinsed and drained
sea salt

Preheat the oven to 350°F. Line a baking tray with baking parchment. Put the oil in a medium bowl and add the lemon zest and juice, paprika, turmeric and ¼ teaspoon salt, then whisk together well.

Add the chickpeas to the bowl and mix well so that they are covered with the spicy oil. Spread the chickpeas over the prepared baking tray and cook 40 minutes, shaking the baking tray occasionally to toss the chickpeas, then returning it to the oven to continue cooking. Serve hot with an extra sprinkling of salt.

   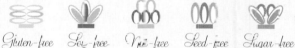

Gluten-free   Soy-free   Nut-free   Seed-free   Sugar-free

cilantro *guacamole*

Serves: 4
Preparation: 15 minutes

3 ripe avocados, cut in half,
   pitted and peeled
juice of ½ lemon
juice of ½ lime
¼ cup finely chopped
   cilantro
¼ onion, finely chopped
1 plum tomato or ripe tomato,
   chopped
½ teaspoon sea salt
¼ teaspoon chili powder
warm sourdough bread or
   corn chips, to serve

Put all the ingredients in a large bowl and mash together using a fork until the mixture is the consistency you'd like—either smooth or with a few lumps for texture. Serve with sourdough bread or corn chips.

Gluten-free   Soy-free   Nut-free   Seed-free   Sugar-free   Raw

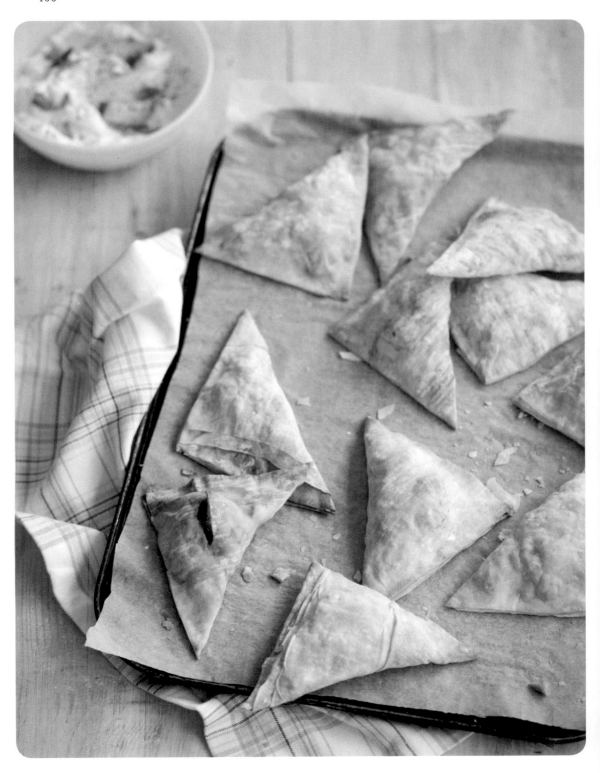

Soy-free   Fat-free   Sugar-free

potato & coconut samosas

Makes: 16 samosas
Preparation: 20 minutes,
plus cooling and making
the relish
Cooking: 30 minutes

⅔ cup cashews
1 tablespoon olive oil or
  coconut oil
½ onion, finely sliced
¾-inch piece fresh ginger
  root, peeled and grated
3 medium potatoes, finely
  chopped
½ teaspoon ground cumin
½ teaspoon ground coriander
¼ cup shredded coconut
3 tablespoons coconut cream
¼ cup chopped cilantro
8 sheets of vegan phyllo
  pastry dough, defrosted
  if frozen
olive oil, for brushing
sea salt and freshly ground
  black pepper
Tomato Relish (page 48),
  hummus or dairy-free
  yogurt with mint, to serve

Preheat the oven to 350°F and line a baking sheet with baking parchment. Put the cashews into a blender or food processor and grind into a powder. Set aside.

Heat the oil in a large nonstick skillet over medium heat, add the onion, ginger and potatoes, and cook 10 minutes, stirring constantly, or until tender.

Stir in the cumin, ground coriander, cashews, shredded coconut, coconut cream and cilantro, then cook another 5 minutes. Season with salt and pepper, then set aside to cool.

Lay the phyllo pastry dough sheets on a clean surface, and brush each one lightly with the oil. Lay one phyllo sheet on top of another and repeat with the remaining sheets to make 4 piles of double-layered phyllo. Cut each pile into four. Put ¼ cup of the mixture into the center of each square, then brush the edges of the phyllo dough with water.

Fold each square into a triangle, then use your fingers to press the edges together. Transfer to the prepared baking sheet. Brush lightly with oil, and bake 15 minutes, or until golden. Serve with your chosen accompaniment.

savory *cookies*

Makes: 25 cookies
Preparation: 15 minutes,
  plus 30 minutes chilling
Cooking: 20 minutes,
  plus cooling

1 cup all-purpose flour, plus
  extra for dusting
¾ teaspoon baking powder
¼ teaspoon sea salt
a large pinch of cayenne
  pepper
¼ teaspoon brown sugar or
  coconut sugar
1 tablespoon nutritional yeast
  flakes
2 tablespoons vegan cream
  cheese
¼ cup olive oil
2 tablespoons soy milk
½ teaspoon wholegrain
  mustard
2 teaspoons caraway seeds
1 tablespoon pumpkin seeds
1 tablespoon sesame seeds
freshly ground black pepper
vegan cheeses and pickles,
  to serve

Sift the flour, baking powder, salt and cayenne pepper into a large bowl, then add the sugar and yeast flakes. Lightly season with black pepper. Stir well to combine.

Put the cream cheese in a small bowl and stir in the oil and milk until the mixture becomes creamy and smooth. Pour into the flour mixture and stir to make a dough, adding up to 1½ tablespoons water, if necessary, to bind. Gather the dough together and put it into a small bowl.

Cover and chill in the refrigerator 30 minutes. Preheat the oven to 350°F and line a baking sheet with baking parchment.

Flour a work surface and roll out the dough to ¼ inch thick, then use a 1¾-inch cookie cutter to cut out circles. Put the mustard in a small bowl and add ½ teaspoon water. Mix together, then brush it over 5 of the cookies. Sprinkle a pinch of caraway seeds over another 5 cookies and do the same with the pumpkin and sesame seeds, then grind some pepper over the remaining cookies. Gently press the seeds and pepper into the dough, then bake 15 to 20 minutes until lightly golden. Carefully transfer the cookies to a wire rack to cool completely before serving. Serve with cheese and pickles. Store in an airtight container up to 3 days.

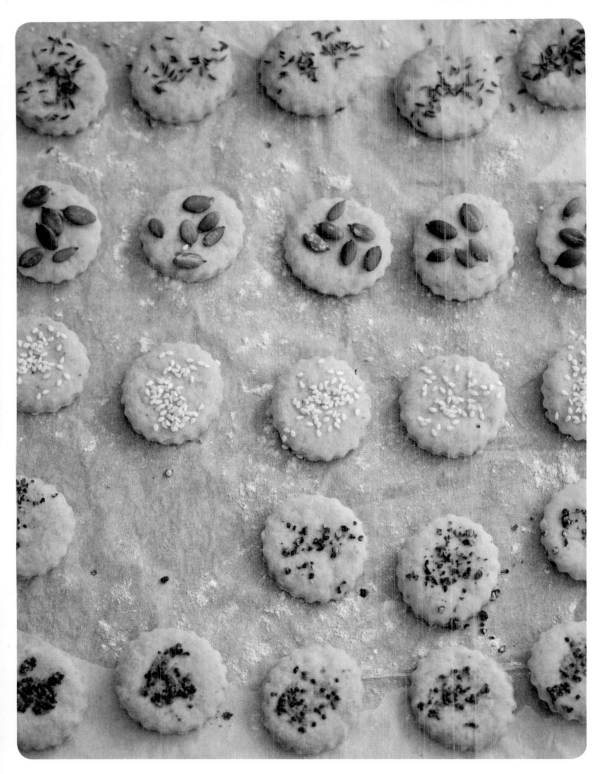

Nut free

chewy chocolate cookies

Makes: 12 cookies
Preparation: 15 minutes,
 plus 10 minutes soaking
Cooking: 15 minutes,
 plus cooling

1 vanilla bean
1 tablespoon chia seeds
1 cup plus 2 tablespoons
 safflower oil, or sunflower
 oil or melted coconut oil
1 cup brown sugar or
 coconut sugar
2½ cups all-purpose flour
1 teaspoon baking powder
½ cup cocoa powder or raw
 cacao powder
5½ ounces vegan dark
 chocolate, chopped into
 small chunks

Preheat the oven to 35C°F and line a baking sheet with baking parchment. Split the vanilla bean in half lengthwise and scrape out the seeds. Reserve the bean for another use. Set the seeds to one side. Put the chia seeds in a small bowl and add 2 tablespoons water. Let soak 10 minutes to form a gel.

Put the oil in the top of a double boiler set over gently simmering water. Add the sugar and whisk together until the sugar has dissolved. Add the vanilla seeds and chia-seed gel. Mix well and set aside.

In a large bowl, sift together the flour, baking powder and cocoa powder. Add the chocolate chunks and stir to combine. Make a small well in the center and add the oil mixture. Stir well. The dough should be soft and not too dry, but firm enough to hold its shape. Add a little water if necessary.

Scoop out a large heaped teaspoonful of the dough and put it on the prepared baking sheet. Use a fork to flatten the dough slightly. Repeat with the remaining dough, spaced evenly apart. Bake 12 to 15 minutes until golden. Let cool on the baking sheet 5 minutes, then transfer to a wire rack to cool completely before serving.

raw sesame *fudge slice*

Makes: 16 squares
Preparation: 5 minutes,
  plus 3 hours chilling

1 cup sesame seeds
½ cup raw cacao powder
2 tablespoons carob powder
scant ½ cup agave syrup or
  brown rice syrup
¼ cup coconut oil, melted

Put the sesame seeds into a blender or food processor and blend until ground. Add the remaining ingredients and blend until well combined. Press into a 12 × 9-inch baking tray and chill in the refrigerator 2 to 3 hours until firm. Cut into squares and serve.

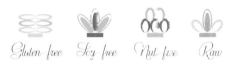

Gluten-free   Soy-free   Nut-free   Raw

quinoa *choc - crackle slice*

Makes: 16 squares
Preparation: 10 minutes,
  plus 2 hours chilling

1½ cups coconut nectar, or
  ½ cup brown sugar or
  coconut sugar
4 cups puffed quinoa
2 tablespoons coconut oil,
  melted
½ teaspoon sea salt
¼ cup almond butter
2 tablespoons raw cacao
  powder or cocoa powder

If using sugar, put it in a small bowl and add ½ cup warm water. Stir to dissolve. Tip the puffed quinoa into a shallow nonstick 9 x 9-inch baking pan and set aside. Put the coconut nectar or sugar-water in a bowl and add the oil, salt, almond butter and cacao powder. Stir well to combine.

Pour this over the puffed quinoa and stir well. Press the mixture down firmly and chill 2 hours. Slice into squares using a sharp knife, then serve. Store in an airtight container up to 2 weeks.

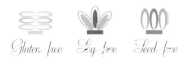

Gluten-free   Soy-free   Seed-free

Rich in triglycerides (medium-chain fatty acids) from the coconut, these bars are perfect for an energy boost. They are also high in vitamin C and healthful flavonoids, and are so tasty that kids (both small and big) will devour them without knowing how healthy they are.

cherry coconut *crunch bars*

Makes: 12 bars
Preparation: 15 minutes,
  plus 30 minutes chilling

2½ cups almonds
⅓ cup chia seeds
½ cup cherries, pitted
¼ cup dried cherries, dried
  cranberries or raisins
½ cup dried medjool dates,
  pitted
¼ cup cacao nibs or chopped
  dark vegan chocolate
¼ cup shredded coconut
1 tablespoon brown sugar or
  coconut sugar
1 tablespoon melted
  coconut oil

Line a 9 × 9-inch baking pan with baking parchment. Put the almonds into a food processor and add the chia seeds, fresh and dried cherries, dates, cacao nibs and shredded coconut. Pulse until the almonds are crushed, then blend on high speed 10 seconds.

Put the sugar in a bowl and add the oil plus scant ⅓ cup warm water. Whisk together until the sugar dissolves. Add to the food processor and blend another 10 seconds, or until combined.

Press the mixture into the prepared pan to a thickness of 1 inch, then chill in the refrigerator 30 minutes or until firm. Cut the mixture into 12 bars and serve. Store in an airtight container in the refrigerator up to 1 week.

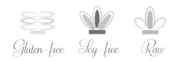

Gluten-free   Soy-free   Raw

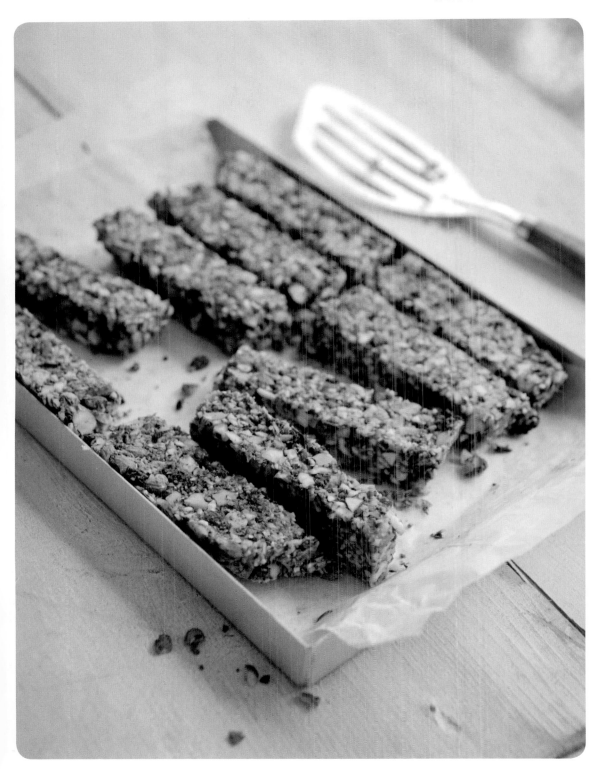

Two of my favorite foods are brought together in these muffins. Chai spices and banana are perfect partners, and are superb when baked in a warm and delicious muffin. Lighter than cake, but denser than cupcakes, these muffins are the best of both worlds.

chai-spiced banana *muffins*

Makes: 12 muffins
Preparation: 15 minutes
Cooking: 25 minutes,
  plus cooling

½ cup coconut milk
1 teaspoon cider vinegar
⅓ cup safflower oil, sunflower oil or melted coconut oil
2 ripe bananas, mashed
1 teaspoon vanilla extract
½ teaspoon ground cardamom
½ teaspoon ground cloves
1 teaspoon ground cinnamon
1 teaspoon ground ginger
½ teaspoon ground allspice
½ teaspoon black pepper
2 cups all-purpose flour
½ teaspoon baking powder
¾ cup pecans, roughly chopped, plus extra to decorate

Preheat the oven to 375°F, and line a 12-cup muffin pan with paper muffin cups. Pour the coconut milk into a small bowl and add the cider vinegar, then whisk together. Set aside.

Put the oil in a large bowl and add the bananas, vanilla extract and spices. Stir well. Sift in half the flour, and the baking powder, and stir in gently, then sift in the remaining flour and briefly stir again. Fold in the pecans.

Divide the mixture evenly into the paper cups and scatter a few chopped pecans over the top. Bake 20 to 25 minutes until firm on top and a skewer inserted into the center comes out clean. Let cool in the pan on a wire rack 5 minutes, then lift out onto the wire rack to cool completely before serving. Store in an airtight container up to 4 days.

Soy free   Sugar-free

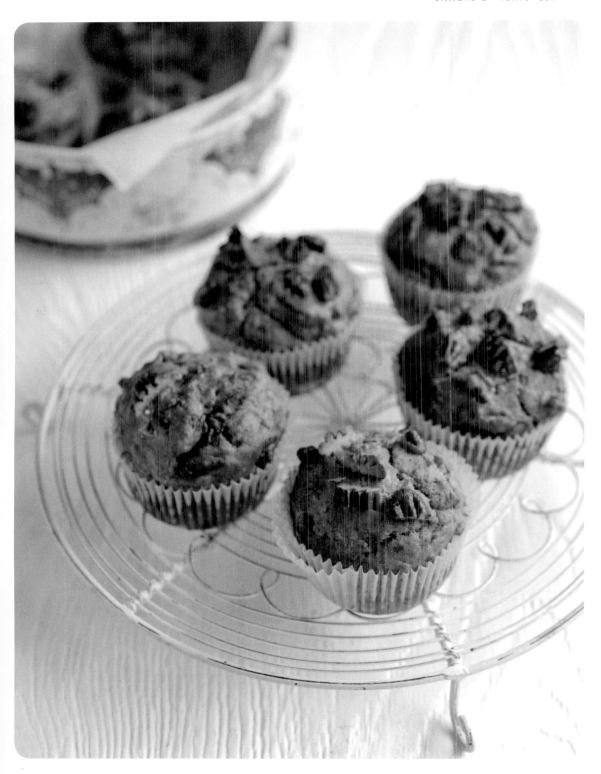

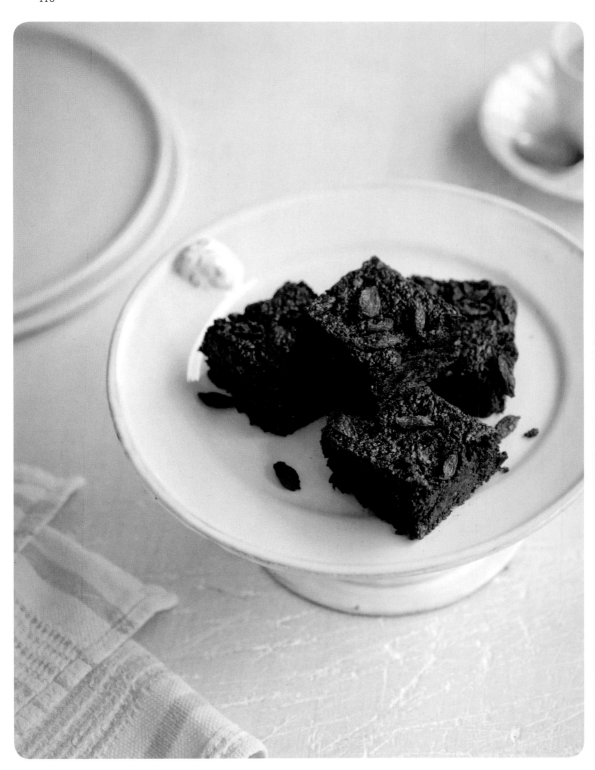

These brownies can be made quickly and easily by just whizzing them up in your blender.

chocolate goji *brownies*

Makes: 12 squares
Preparation: 5 minutes,
  plus 5 minutes soaking
Cooking: 45 minutes,
  plus cooling

½ cup goji berries, dried
  dates or apricots, chopped,
  plus extra to decorate
  (optional)
1 vanilla bean
1 cup gluten-free flour blend
1 teaspoon sea salt
¾ cup cocoa powder or raw
  cacao powder
½ cup brown sugar or
  coconut sugar
¾ cup safflower oil, sunflower
  oil or melted coconut oil
¼ cup ground flaxseed

Preheat the oven to 350°F Put the goji berries in a small bowl and cover with water. Let soak 5 minutes, then drain in a colander. Split the vanilla bean in half lengthwise and scrape out the seeds. Reserve the bean for another use.

Sift the flour, salt and cocoa powder into a food processor and add the sugar and vanilla seeds. Blend on high speed 20 seconds. (Alternatively, put the ingredients in a mixing bowl and stir thoroughly.) Add the oil, ground flaxseed, goji berries and 2 tablespoons water, then blend 20 seconds, or stir well, until combined.

Pour the mixture into a 9 x 9-inch nonstick baking pan. Scatter with extra fruit, if using, and cook 40 to 45 minutes until a skewer inserted into the center comes out clean. Let cool, then cut into 12 squares before serving. Store in an airtight container up to 1 week.

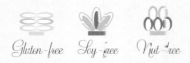

Gluten-free   *Soy-free*   *Nut-free*

lime & coconut *cupcakes*

Makes: 14 cupcakes
Preparation: 30 minutes, plus
** making the optional milk**
Cooking: 20 minutes, plus
** cooling**

1¾ cups all-purpose flour
2 teaspoons baking powder
a pinch of sea salt
¾ cup brown sugar or
  coconut sugar
⅓ cup shredded coconut,
  plus extra to decorate
1 cup plus 2 tablespoons
  coconut milk or Almond
  Milk (page 20)
½ cup safflower oil or
  sunflower oil
1 teaspoon almond extract
1 teaspoon vanilla paste
1 tablespoon cider vinegar

FROSTING
⅓ cup vegan margarine
4 teaspoons Almond Milk
finely grated zest of 1 lime,
  plus extra to decorate
½ teaspoon lime juice
2 cups powdered sugar

Preheat the oven to 350°F and line 14 muffin cups with paper cups. Sift the flour, baking powder and salt into a large bowl and stir in the sugar and coconut. Pour the milk into a separate bowl and add the oil, almond extract, vanilla paste and vinegar. Mix well, then pour the milk mixture into the dry ingredients and stir with a wooden spoon until just combined.

Divide the mixture into the paper cups until three-quarters full. Bake 18 minutes, or until well risen and a skewer inserted into the center of a cupcake comes out clean. Remove the cupcakes from the pan and transfer them to a wire rack to cool completely.

To make the frosting, put the margarine, milk, lime zest and juice in a large mixing bowl and sift in the powdered sugar. Beat, using a whisk or an electric beater, until light and fluffy. Swirl the frosting onto the top of each cupcake. Top with a sprinkling of coconut and lime zest, and serve.

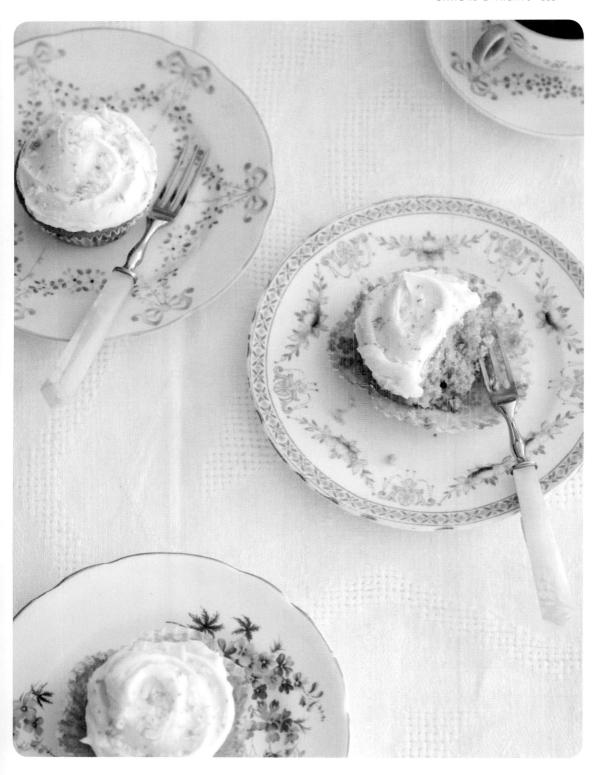

Soy-free

spiced apple *tea cake*

Serves: 8–10
Preparation: 15 minutes,
  plus 10 minutes soaking
  and making the milk
Cooking: 1¼ hours, plus
  cooling

2 tablespoons chia seeds
scant ⅔ cup safflower oil,
  sunflower oil or melted
  coconut oil, plus extra for
  greasing
1½ cups all-purpose flour
2 teaspoons baking powder
1½ tablespoons ground
  ginger
1 teaspoon ground cinnamon
1 cup brown sugar or
  coconut sugar
¼ cup Almond Milk
  (page 20)

APPLE TOPPING
1 cup brown sugar or
  coconut sugar
grated zest and juice of
  1 lemon
1 teaspoon ground cinnamon
2 eating apples, peeled,
  cored and thinly sliced

Put the chia seeds in a small bowl and add ¼ cup water. Let soak 10 minutes to form a gel. Preheat the oven to 350°F and lightly grease a 9-inch cake pan.

To make the apple topping, pour 3¼ cups water into a small saucepan over medium heat and add the sugar, lemon zest and juice, and the cinnamon. Stir gently, then bring to a gentle boil, and add the apple slices. Cook 10 minutes, or until the apples are tender but still holding their shape, then remove from the liquid using a slotted spoon. Set the apples aside to cool, discarding the cooking liquid.

Meanwhile, sift the flour, baking powder, ginger and cinnamon into a large mixing bowl and stir in the sugar. Pour the oil into the bowl with the chia-seed gel and add ¼ cup water and the milk. Mix together well, then pour this mixture into the dry ingredients in the mixing bowl. Stir until just incorporated, but do not over-mix.

Tip the batter into the prepared pan and level the top. Lay the apple slices on the top, starting at the outside edge and working into the center. Bake 55 minutes, or until the cake springs back when pressed. Let cool in the pan on a wire rack, then remove from the pan and serve.

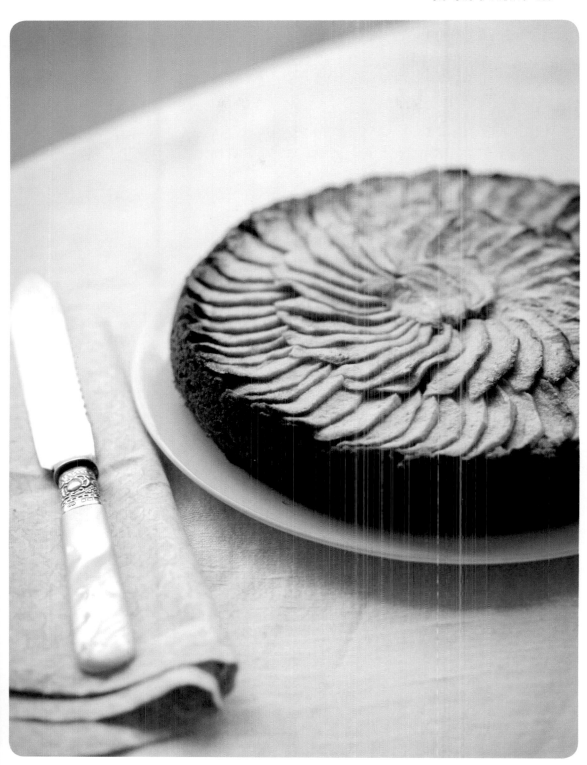

This beautiful, richly flavored loaf takes very little time to prepare using your blender.

almond & coconut loaf

Makes: 1 loaf (10 slices)
Preparation: 10 minutes,
  plus 10 minutes soaking,
  and making the milk and
  optional spread
Cooking: 1 hour, plus cooling

1 tablespoon chia seeds
1 cup safflower oil, or
  sunflower oil or melted
  coconut oil, plus extra for
  greasing
grated zest of 1 orange
¾ cup brown sugar or
  coconut sugar
3 cups all-purpose flour
2 teaspoons baking powder
1 cup shredded coconut
⅔ cup ground almonds
1 cup plus 2 tablespoons
  Almond Milk (page 20)
berries or Fruit & Pumpkin
  Spread (page 26), to serve

Put the chia seeds in a small bowl and add 3 tablespoons water. Let soak 10 minutes to form a gel. Preheat the oven to 350°F, and grease a 8½ x 4½-inch loaf pan.

Put the oil in a blender or food processor and add the orange zest and sugar. Add the chia-seed gel and blend until mixed. Sift in the flour and baking powder and add the coconut, ground almonds and milk, then blend on high speed 30 seconds, or until combined.

Pour into the prepared loaf pan and bake 1 hour, or until the loaf springs back when pressed. Let the loaf cool in the pan, then turn it onto a wire rack. Serve with fresh berries or a large spoonful of spread. Store in an airtight container up to 1 week.

Soy-free

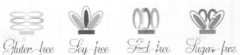

Gluten-free Soy-free Egg-free Sugar-free

peach, orange blossom &
coconut popsicles

Makes: 6 popsicles
Preparation: 5 minutes,
  plus 20 minutes soaking
  and 4 hours freezing, and
  making the milk

2 fresh or dried medjool
  dates, pitted
4 large peaches, cut in half,
  pitted and chopped
¾ cup plus 2 tablespoons
  coconut milk
¾ cup plus 2 tablespoons
  Almond Milk (page 20)
1 teaspoon orange
  blossom water

If using dried dates, put them in a small bowl and cover with water. Let soak 20 minutes then drain in a colander.

Put all the ingredients into a blender or food processor and blend until smooth. Pour the mixture into 6 popsicle molds and freeze 3 to 4 hours until firm. Serve.

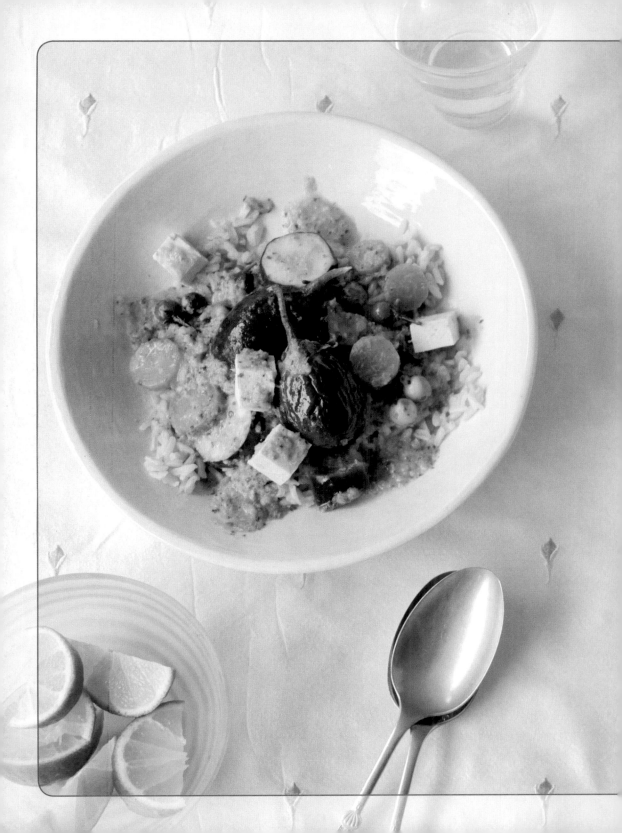

Main Meals

The main meal of the day is a chance for couples or families to sit together and chat over their favorite dishes—steamy bowls of robust soups, homemade burgers and spicy curries. There's nothing better than to fill up on a wholesome dish that doesn't feel heavy on the stomach, and these plant-based recipes certainly fit the bill. Quinoa Stuffed Peppers are spicy and have a sweet and nutty edge, Moussaka with Cottage-Feta Cheese is based on vegetables rather than pasta, and South African Sweet Potato Stew is spicy and warming. You'll find noodle and risotto dishes as well as an appealing Rustic Tart with Spinach Pesto—and you can save any leftovers for lunch tomorrow.

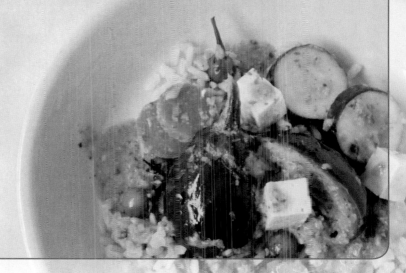

Thai Green Eggplant Curry (page 134).

This is a fast and easy main-course soup that looks and tastes inviting. Make it smooth or leave it crunchy.

chili peanut & coconut soup

Serves: 4
Preparation: 15 minutes
Cooking: 35 minutes

7 ounces tempeh, cubed
2 tablespoons tamari soy
 sauce or soy sauce
2 teaspoons crushed chilies
2 tablespoons toasted
 sesame oil
1 onion, finely chopped
1 red bell pepper, seeded
 and chopped
3 garlic cloves, crushed
1 small red chili, seeded and
 finely chopped
1 cup unsalted roasted
 peanuts, roughly chopped,
 plus 2 tablespoons chopped
 peanuts, to serve
1¾ cups coconut milk
4 scallions, thinly sliced
scant 2 cups bean sprouts
1 small handful snow peas
 or green beans, sliced
 diagonally
1 handful of cilantro
cooked brown rice or nan
 bread, to serve

Put the tempeh in a large bowl and add 1 tablespoon of the tamari and the crushed chilies. Toss well. Heat 1 tablespoon of the oil in a heavy saucepan over medium heat and cook the tempeh 5 minutes, or until golden brown, turning regularly. Remove and set aside. Heat the remaining oil in the pan and add the onion, pepper and garlic. Cook 5 to 8 minutes until softened. Add the chili and roasted peanuts, and stir constantly 2 minutes, until fragrant.

Add the remaining tamari, 2½ cups water, and the coconut milk, and bring the soup gently to a boil. Lower the heat, and simmer 15 minutes, or until the soup thickens slightly.

If you prefer a smooth soup, use a blender to puree it to your preferred consistency. Divide into bowls, and add the tempeh, scallions, bean sprouts, snow peas and cilantro, then sprinkle some chopped peanuts over the top. Serve with brown rice.

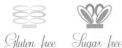

Gluten-free *Sugar-free*

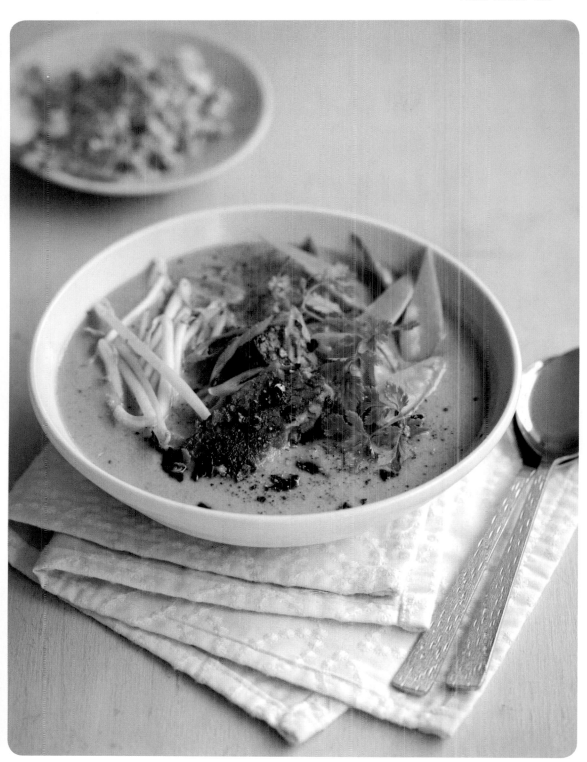

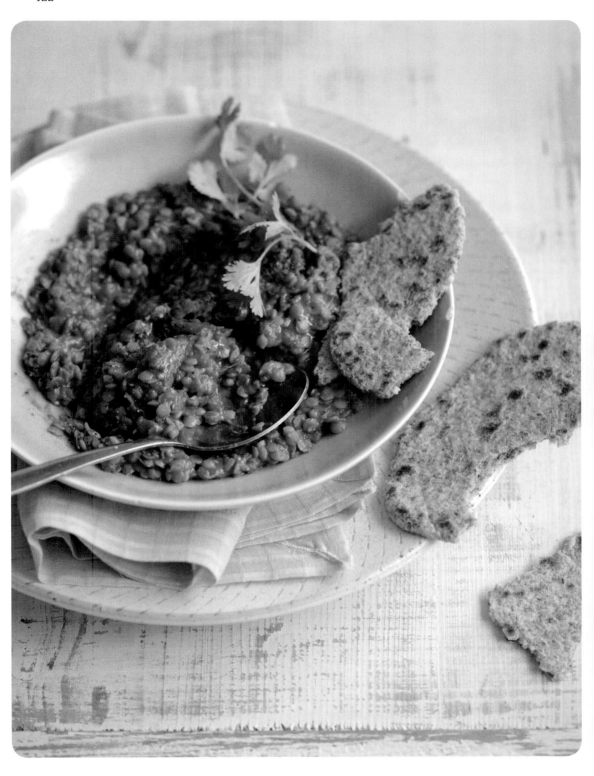

I have made a number of tweaks to this recipe over the years to give it a more complex flavor. Coconut cream is a staple ingredient in Asian dishes and is a wonderful way to add richness and depth.

coconut & red lentil dal

Serves: 4
Preparation: 15 minutes,
 plus making the parathas
Cooking: 45 minutes

1 tablespoon olive oil or
 coconut oil
1 large onion, chopped
3 garlic cloves, crushed
½-inch piece fresh ginger
 root, peeled and grated
2 teaspoons cumin seeds
1 teaspoon yellow mustard
 seeds
2 teaspoons garam masala
1 teaspoon ground turmeric
2 teaspoons dried fenugreek
 leaves
1 teaspoon ground cumin
1 teaspoon ground coriander
1 teaspoon crushed chilies
 (optional)
1 cup red lentils, rinsed and
 drained
1¾ cups coconut cream
2 cups canned chopped
 tomatoes
1 teaspoon sea salt
juice of 1 lime
fresh cilantro and Garlic
 Parathas (page 27) or
 cooked brown rice, to serve

Heat the oil in a large saucepan over medium-high heat and add the onion and garlic. Cook 5 to 8 minutes, stirring frequently, until softened. Add the ginger, cumin seeds and mustard seeds, and cook another 2 minutes, or until the seeds begin to pop. Add 1 tablespoon water, if the mixture is sticking to the pan, and then add the garam masala, turmeric, fenugreek, ground cumin, coriander and crushed chilies, f using. Stir until the mixture forms a thick, brown paste.

Add the lentils, coconut cream, tomatoes and 1 cup water. Bring to a boil, then reduce the heat to a simmer and cook 20 minutes, stirring frequently. Add the salt and lime juice, and cook 10 minutes more. Serve with a sprig of cilantro and parathas.

Gluten-free *Soy-free* *Seed-free* *Sugar-free*

pan-fried sage & *basil gnocchi*

Serves: 4
Preparation: 15 minutes,
  plus 10 minutes resting
  and making the cheese
Cooking: 45 minutes

1 pound, 2 ounces baking
  potatoes, such as Idaho or
  russet, cubed
1½ cups all-purpose flour,
  plus extra if needed and
  for dusting
1 tablespoon finely chopped
  sage leaves
1 tablespoon finely chopped
  basil leaves
1 tablespoon safflower oil or
  sunflower oil
1 cup pitted mixed green and
  black olives, chopped
1 red chili, seeded and thinly
  sliced lengthwise
2 cups baby spinach leaves
½ cup drained sun-dried
  tomatoes in oil, chopped
7 ounces bottled or canned
  artichoke hearts
1 handful of basil leaves, torn
7 ounces Herbed Almond
  Cheese (page 22), crumbled
sea salt and freshly ground
  black pepper

Put the potatoes in a steamer set over a pan of boiling water and steam over medium heat 15 to 20 minutes until soft. Preheat the oven to 200°F and put a baking tray inside to warm.

Put the potatoes in a bowl, mash them and sift in 1¼ cups flour, the herbs and add a good pinch of salt. Mix by hand until just combined, adding the remaining flour. Turn the dough onto a floured surface and knead 1 minute. If the dough is sticky, add more flour, 1 teaspoon at a time, until the dough is soft and workable. Let it rest 10 minutes.

Bring a large pot of salted water to a boil over high heat, then reduce to medium-high. Divide the dough into four pieces and roll them into long sausage shapes. Slice each piece into ¾-inch pieces to make gnocchi. Lower the gnocchi in batches into the boiling water using a slotted spoon, and cook 5 minutes, or until they float to the surface. Remove from the pot as they cook and lay them on the baking tray and keep them warm while you cook the remaining gnocchi.

Heat the oil in a large, nonstick skillet over medium-high heat and fry the gnocchi in batches, keeping the cooked gnocchi warm on the tray. Add the olives and chili to the skillet, and cook 5 minutes. Add the spinach, followed by the tomatoes, artichokes and basil. Return the gnocchi to the skillet and gently toss with the vegetables. Season with pepper and serve topped with the herbed cheese.

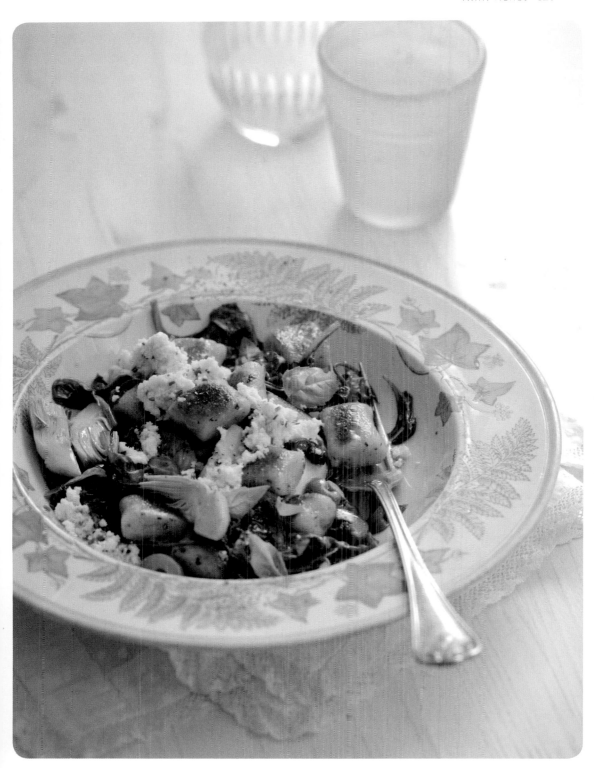

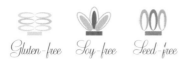

Gluten-free Soy-free Seed-free Sugar-free

quinoa stuffed peppers

Serves: 4
Preparation: 15 minutes, plus
10 minutes soaking and
making the sauce
Cooking: 1 hour 5 minutes

2 fresh or dried medjool
  dates, pitted and chopped
4 red bell peppers
1 tablespoon olive oil or
  coconut oil
1 onion, chopped
1 garlic clove, crushed
1 teaspoon ground turmeric
¼ teaspoon ground
  cinnamon
1 teaspoon cumin seeds
½ teaspoon ground
  cardamom
½ cup red quinoa, rinsed and
  drained
½ cup white quinoa, rinsed
  and drained
3 cups canned chickpeas,
  rinsed and drained
1 dried fig, finely chopped
4 ready-to-eat dried apricots,
  finely chopped
1 large handful of cilantro,
  chopped
3 tablespoons pine nuts
sea salt
Chermoula Sauce (page 85),
  to serve

Preheat the oven to 350°F and line a baking tray or ovenproof dish with baking parchment. If using dried dates, put the chopped dates in a small bowl and cover with water. Let soak 10 minutes, then drain in a strainer.

Cut the peppers in half through the stalk and remove the seeds and pith from inside. Set the peppers to one side.

Heat the oil in a nonstick skillet over medium heat. Fry the onion and garlic 7 to 8 minutes until beginning to soften, then add the turmeric, cinnamon, cumin seeds and cardamom. Set aside.

Meanwhile, pour 2 cups boiling water into a medium saucepan over high heat and add both types of quinoa. Boil 15 minutes, or until tender and translucent. Drain the quinoa in a strainer and rinse, then drain thoroughly and tip into a large bowl. Stir in the onion mixture, the chickpeas, fig, dates, apricots, cilantro and pine nuts. Season with salt.

Spoon into the peppers and bake 30 to 40 minutes until tender. Serve with chermoula sauce.

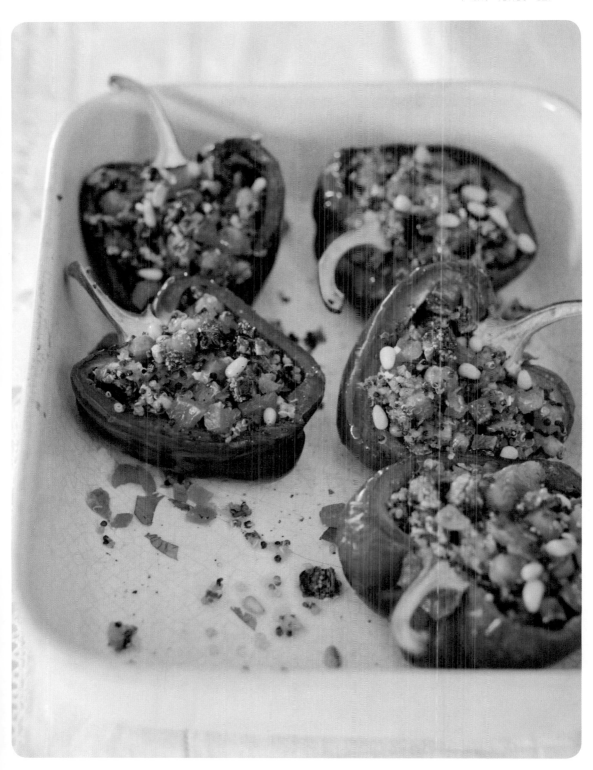

While in Thailand, I learned that the essence of Thai food is in the balance of sweetness, saltiness, spiciness and sourness—I have aimed for that perfect relationship here.

khao soi–thai curry noodles

Serves: 4
Preparation: 15 minutes, plus
  making the curry paste
Cooking: 20 minutes

1 tablespoon toasted
  sesame oil
1 cup cashews
2 tablespoons Thai Red Curry
  Paste (page 25)
2 zucchini, cut in half
  and sliced
1 carrot, chopped
14 ounces button mushrooms,
  sliced
2½ tablespoons tomato paste
1¾ cups canned coconut
  milk
2 teaspoons curry powder
3 tablespoons tamari soy
  sauce or soy sauce
2 teaspoons brown sugar or
  coconut sugar
5½ ounces rice vermicelli
  noodles
1 cup bean sprouts, plus
  extra to serve
¼ cup cilantro
4 scallions, diagonally sliced
lime wedges, to serve

Heat the sesame oil in a large saucepan over medium-high heat. Add the cashews and cook 3 to 4 minutes, stirring regularly, until golden brown. Remove the nuts from the pan and drain on paper towels. Set aside. Reduce the heat to medium.

Add the curry paste to the pan and stir constantly 30 seconds, or until fragrant. Add the zucchini, carrot, mushrooms and tomato paste, and stir well. Pour in the coconut milk and 2 cups water, the curry powder, tamari and sugar, and bring gently to a boil. Reduce the heat and simmer 10 minutes, or until the carrot is tender.

Meanwhile, put the vermicelli noodles in a heatproof bowl and pour in boiling water to cover generously. Gently move the noodles in the water, using a fork, and leave 5 to 6 minutes until soft.

Add the bean sprouts to the vegetable mixture just before serving, stir well and remove from the heat. Drain the noodles in a colander and divide into four large serving bowls. Ladle the soup and vegetables over the noodles, and top with the fried cashews, cilantro, scallions and extra bean sprouts. Serve with the wedges of lime.

Gluten-free

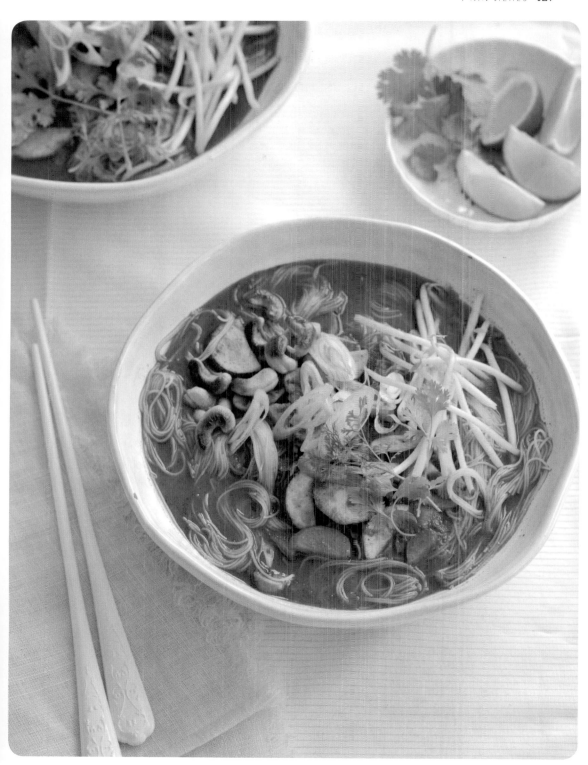

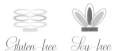
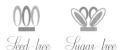

Gluten-free   Soy-free   Seed-free   Sugar-free

moussaka with cottage-feta cheese

Serves: 4
Preparation: 30 minutes,
   plus making the cheese
Cooking: 1 hour 15 minutes

4 tablespoons olive oil or
   coconut oil, plus extra for
   greasing
1 large eggplant, thinly
   sliced
2 zucchini, thinly sliced
   lengthwise
2 potatoes, thinly sliced
1 onion, chopped
2 garlic cloves, crushed
4 cups canned chopped
   tomatoes
1 cup White Cottage-Feta
   Cheese (page 21), crumbled
1 cup canned brown lentils,
   rinsed and drained
2 cups tomato sauce
sea salt and freshly ground
   black pepper
green salad and olives,
   to serve

Preheat the oven to 400°F, and lightly grease a 9 × 13-inch baking dish. Heat 1 tablespoon of the oil in a nonstick skillet over medium heat. Working in batches, lightly brown the eggplant, zucchini and potatoes on both sides, adding more oil as necessary. As each batch finishes, transfer to a colander lined with paper towels and let drain.

Meanwhile, heat the remaining oil in a saucepan and cook the onion and garlic for 5 to 8 minutes until softened, then stir in the tomatoes and bring to a boil. Season with salt and pepper, and cook 5 minutes.

Place a layer of eggplant, zucchini and potatoes in the prepared baking dish and top with ¼ cup of the tomato mixture, then scatter ¼ cup of cheese and ¼ cup of lentils over it. Season lightly with salt and pepper. Pour over enough tomato sauce for a light covering.

Make 3 more layers in the same way, pressing the layers down firmly. Add all the remaining tomato sauce to the top layer. Bake 35 minutes, or until thoroughly heated through and bubbling at the sides. Serve with a big green salad and plenty of olives.

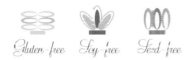

Gluten-free Soy-free Seed-free

baked polenta with tomato &
basil sauce

Serves: 4
Preparation: 15 minutes
Cooking: 1 hour

1 tablespoon plus 1 teaspoon
   olive oil or coconut oil, plus
   extra for greasing
1 cup polenta
¼ cup ground almonds
4⅓ cups vegetable stock
2 tablespoons lemon juice
½ cup pine nuts
1 onion, chopped
1 garlic clove, crushed
2 cups canned chopped
   tomatoes
1 handful of basil leaves,
   plus 1 tablespoon chopped
   basil leaves
1 teaspoon dried oregano
½ teaspoon crushed chilies
½ teaspoon brown sugar or
   coconut sugar
sea salt and freshly ground
   black pepper

Preheat the oven to 350°F and lightly grease a 2-quart shallow baking dish. Put the polenta and ground almonds in a bowl and add the stock, a pinch of salt and the lemon juice. Stir well to combine, then pour it into the baking dish and spread out evenly (the ground almonds will float to the top and the polenta will sink to the bottom). Bake 45 minutes.

Meanwhile, put the pine nuts in a large saucepan over medium heat and dry-toast 1 to 2 minutes or until golden, shaking the pan frequently. Tip onto a small plate and set aside.

Add 1 tablespoon of the oil to the pan and add the onion and garlic, and cook 5 to 8 minutes until softened. Add the tomatoes, 1 tablespoon chopped basil, the oregano, crushed chilies and sugar, and add enough water to just cover. Season with salt and pepper, and bring to a gentle boil, then reduce the heat and simmer 15 minutes.

Remove the semi-set polenta from the oven and stir in the 1 teaspoon oil. If using coconut oil, this will melt immediately. Bake another 15 minutes or until crisp on top. The ground almonds will create a delicious crust. Spoon the tomato sauce over the polenta and scatter the toasted pine nuts and the basil leaves over the top. Add a grinding of black pepper and serve.

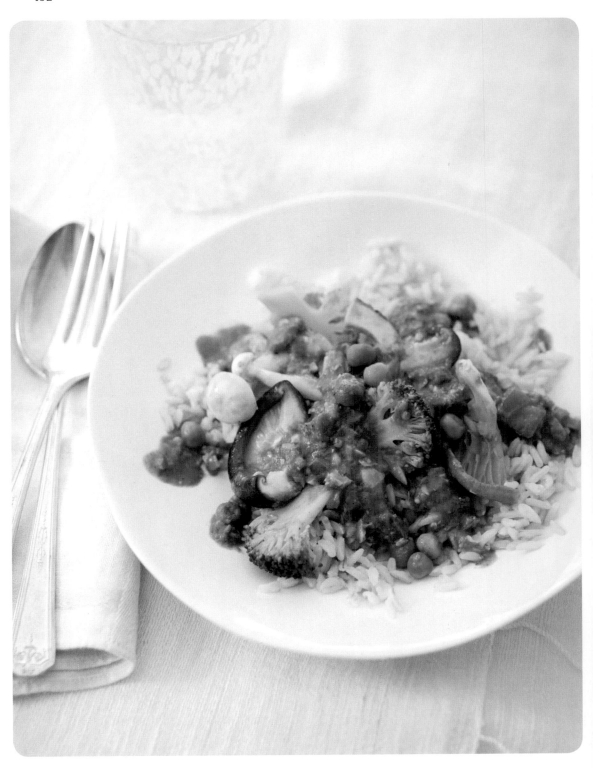

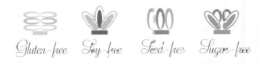

Gluten-free Soy-free Seed-free Sugar-free

mushroom & pea coconut korma

Serves: 4
Preparation: 15 minutes,
  plus making the optional
  parathas
Cooking: 1 hour

1 teaspoon olive oil or
  coconut oil
1 onion, chopped
3 garlic cloves, crushed
1 teaspoon cumin seeds
1 teaspoon yellow mustard
  seeds
2 teaspoons garam masala
1 tablespoon ground turmeric
1 tablespoon dried fenugreek
  leaves
7 ounces mixed mushrooms,
  sliced or cut in half, if large
1½ cups coconut milk
2 cups canned chopped
  tomatoes
7 ounces tomatoes, chopped
4 ounces broccoli florets, cut
  in half
1 cup shelled green peas or
  frozen peas
1 cup almonds, roughly
  chopped
cooked brown rice, quinoa or
  Garlic Parathas (page 27),
  to serve

Heat the oil in a large saucepan over medium heat and add the onion and garlic. Cook 5 to 8 minutes until softened. Add the cumin seeds and mustard seeds, and stir-fry 30 seconds, or until they begin to pop. Add the garam masala, turmeric and fenugreek, and stir to combine

Add the mushrooms, coconut milk, ½ cup water and the canned and fresh tomatoes, then stir and bring to a gentle boil, stirring frequently. Cook over medium-low heat 20 minutes, or until the mushrooms are soft and the sauce has thickened. Add the broccoli and peas and cook another 10 minutes. Stir in the chopped almonds just before serving. Serve with brown rice.

There are three types of eggplant used in this fragrant dish. You should be able to find them in an Asian grocer's or market, but if not, you can substitute them with 1 pound regular eggplants, cut into cubes.

thai green eggplant curry

Serves: 4
Preparation: 10 minutes, plus
  making the curry paste
Cooking: 20 minutes

1 teaspoon olive oil or
  coconut oil
3 tablespoons Thai Green
  Curry Paste (page 25)
1¾ cups coconut milk
4 ounces eggplant, cubed
  (1 cup)
9 ounces baby eggplants
1 cup pea eggplants, or baby
  eggplants cut into quarters
1 carrot, thinly sliced
1 zucchini, sliced
½ teaspoon tamari soy sauce
  or soy sauce, or to taste
1 teaspoon brown sugar or
  coconut sugar, or to taste
12 ounces firm tofu, cubed
2 tablespoons fresh lime juice
2 kaffir lime leaves, torn
sea salt
cooked brown rice, to serve

Heat the oil in a large pot over medium heat and add the curry paste. Cook 1 minute, stirring frequently, until fragrant.

Add the coconut milk, 1 cup water, all the eggplants, the carrot and zucchini, and bring gently to a boil. Reduce the heat, and add the tamari and sugar. Season with salt. Adjust those three seasonings to taste, to balance the salty-spicy-sour-sweet flavors.

Add the tofu and simmer 10 minutes. Add the lime juice and kaffir lime leaves, then serve over brown rice.

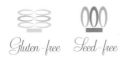

Gluten-free   *Seed-free*

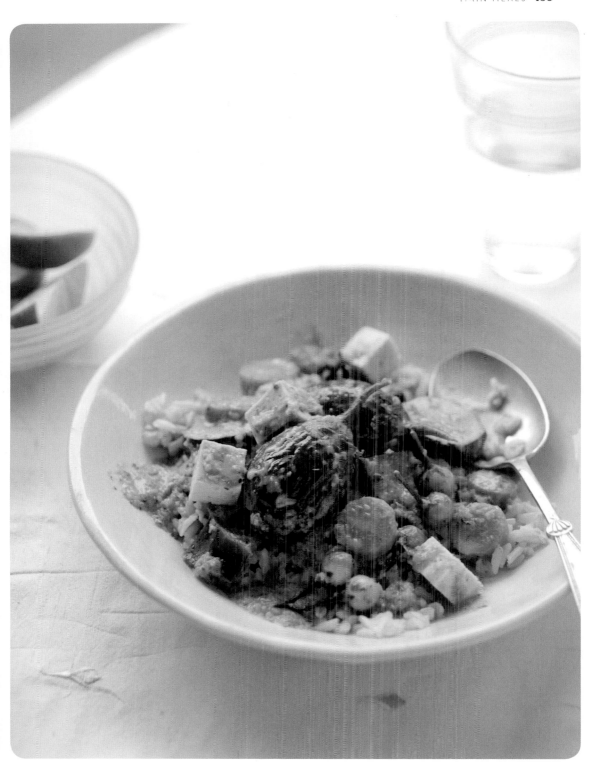

Traditionally a Hare Krishna dish, this curry is so simple to make, and it tastes good and is inexpensive.

curried cabbage with *potatoes*

Serves: 4
Preparation: 15 minutes,
  plus making the dal
  and parathas
Cooking: 25 minutes

2 tablespoons plus
  2 teaspoons olive oil
  or coconut oil
¾ cup peanuts
2 tablespoons curry powder
3 large potatoes, unpeeled
  and cubed
1 garlic clove, crushed
½-inch piece fresh ginger
  root, peeled and grated
1 teaspoon garam masala
½ teaspoon ground turmeric
½ teaspoon brown sugar or
  coconut sugar
1 pound green cabbage,
  thinly sliced
1¼ cups canned chopped
  tomatoes
¾ cup vegetable stock
sea salt
Coconut & Red Lentil Dal
  (page 123) and Garlic
  Parathas (page 27), to serve

Heat 2 teaspoons of the oil in a large skillet over medium-high heat and add the peanuts and curry powder. Mix together well and cook 5 minutes, stirring frequently. Remove the spicy peanuts from the skillet and set aside.

Heat the remaining oil in the same skillet and add the potatoes. Cook 10 minutes, stirring frequently to ensure they don't stick to the bottom, or until lightly golden brown and partly cooked. Remove from the skillet and set aside.

Add the garlic, ginger, garam masala, turmeric and sugar to the skillet. Stir quickly, to release the flavors, then add the cabbage. Stir to coat, then return the potatoes to the skillet followed by the tomatoes and stock. Season with salt.

Reduce the heat to low, cover the skillet and simmer gently 10 minutes, or until the cabbage is tender and the potatoes are cooked through. Top with the spicy peanuts and serve with dal and parathas.

Gluten-free   *Soy-free*   *Seed-free*

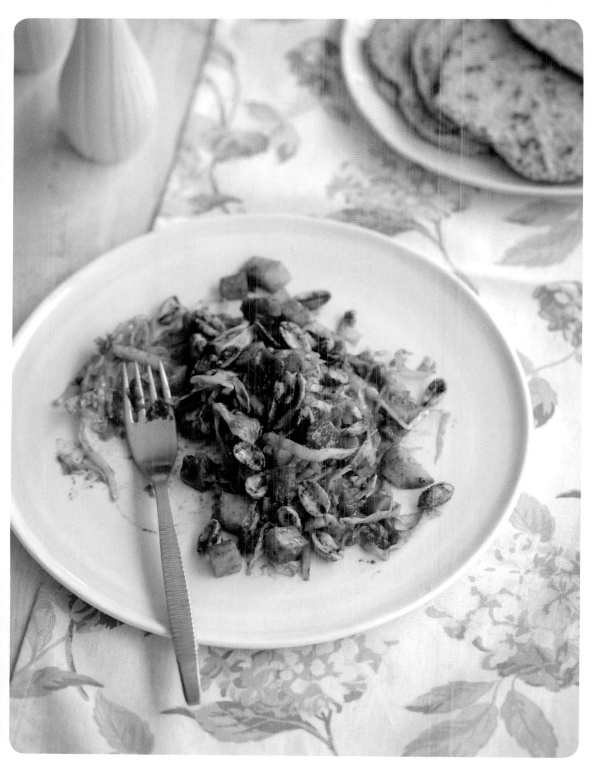

This hearty dish is flavored with ginger, and the peanut butter gives it richness.

south african sweet potato stew

Serves: 4
Preparation: 15 minutes
Cooking: 50 minutes

2 teaspoons olive oil or coconut oil
4 garlic cloves, crushed
1 red bell pepper, seeded and cubed
1 teaspoon crushed chilies
½ teaspoon ground cinnamon
1 teaspoon ground ginger
1 teaspoon brown sugar or coconut sugar
11 ounces sweet potato, cubed
2 cups canned chopped tomatoes
1 cup vegetable stock
2 teaspoons tomato paste
1 tablespoon peanut butter
2½ cups canned red kidney beans, rinsed and drained
2 tablespoons chopped cilantro
sea salt and freshly ground black pepper
cooked brown rice, to serve

Heat the oil in a large, nonstick pot over medium heat and add the garlic and pepper. Cook 10 minutes, or until tender. Add the spices and stir until fragrant.

Add the sugar, sweet potato, tomatoes, stock, tomato paste and peanut butter, and stir well. Bring gently to a boil, then reduce the heat and simmer 25 minutes, or until the sweet potato is tender.

Add the kidney beans and cook another 10 minutes, adding more water, 1 tablespoon at a time, if the mixture looks a little dry. Season with salt and pepper. Scatter the cilantro over it and serve with brown rice.

Gluten-free

Soy-free

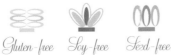
Seed-free

The whole family will enjoy this hearty meal and everyone can prepare their own burritos. Serve with ice tea.

spicy mexican *burritos*

Serves: 4
**Preparation: 15 minutes, plus
making the optional cheese
and guacamole**
**Cooking: 40 minutes, plus
cooling**

1 cup brown rice
2 cups canned red kidney
   beans, rinsed and drained
2 garlic cloves, crushed
2 cups tomato sauce
2 plum tomatoes, chopped
1 tablespoon tomato paste
1 teaspoon ground cumin
1 teaspoon ground turmeric
1 teaspoon chili powder
juice of 1 lemon
juice of 1 lime
1 large handful of cilantro,
   finely chopped
1 large handful of parsley
   leaves, finely chopped
8 flour tortillas
3 cups mixed salad greens,
   plus extra to serve
4 ounces Herbed Almond
   Cheese (optional) (page 22),
   plus extra to serve
Cilantro Guacamole
   (page 99), to serve
sea salt

Pour 2 cups boiling water into a large saucepan, add a pinch of salt and the rice, and return to a boil. Cook 35 to 40 minutes, or according to the rice package instructions, until tender. Drain in a colander and set aside to cool slightly.

Put the kidney beans in a medium saucepan over medium heat and add the garlic, tomato sauce, tomatoes, tomato paste, cumin, turmeric and chili powder. Mix together well. Bring gently to a boil then remove from the heat. Set to one side to cool slightly.

Put the cooked brown rice in a bowl and add the lemon and lime juice, cilantro and parsley. Mix well.

To make the burritos, put 1 tablespoon rice mixture on a tortilla, top with 1 tablespoon kidney beans and then add some salad greens and cheese, if using. Roll up the tortilla, tucking in the bottom edge and leaving the top open. Serve with cheese, if you like, guacamole and salad.

Soy-free

Nut-free

Seed-free

Sugar-free

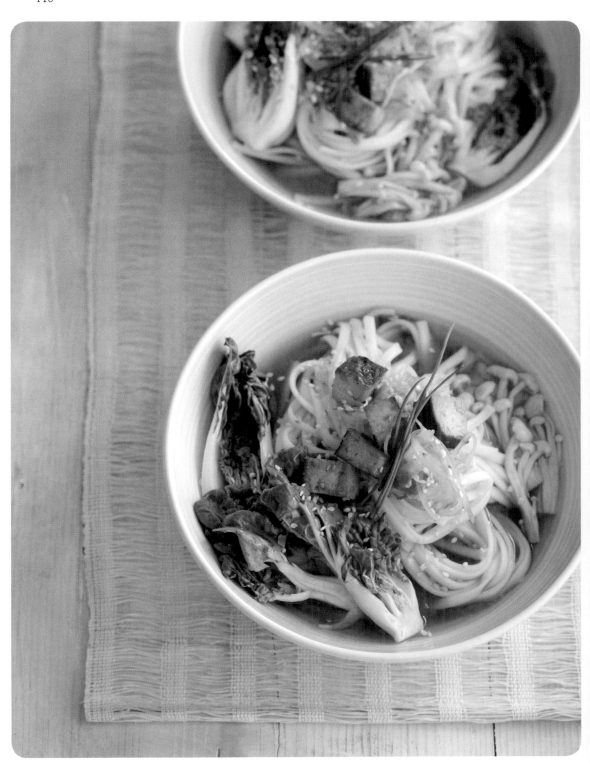

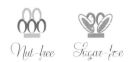

Nut-free   Sugar-free

udon noodle bowl

Serves: 4
Preparation: 15 minutes
Cooking: 25 minutes

12 ounces udon noodles
3 tablespoons toasted
  sesame oil
14 ounces firm smoked tofu,
  cubed
2 tablespoons sesame seeds
1 cup sliced shallots
2 teaspoons rice vinegar
2 teaspoons mirin or rice
  wine vinegar
2 tablespoons miso
8 bok choy, cut in half
  lengthwise
1½ cups enoki mushrooms,
  trimmed, or baby button
  mushrooms, cut in half
sea salt
12 chives, whole or chopped,
  to serve

Bring a large pot of salted water to a boil over high heat.
Add the noodles and cook 8 to 10 minutes, or according to
the package instructions, until tender. Drain in a colander, rinse
with cold water and drain again, then set aside. Meanwhile,
heat 1 tablespoon of the oil in a small skillet over medium-high
heat and fry the tofu 5 to 10 minutes, turning occasionally,
until golden on all sides.

While the tofu fries, heat a wok or large pot over medium heat.
Add the sesame seeds and dry-fry 2 to 3 minutes, stirring
continuously, until just beginning to brown. Tip the sesame seeds
onto a plate and set aside

Pour the remaining oil into the wok and add the shallots. Fry
2 to 5 minutes until softened. Add the rice vinegar, mirin and
miso, and tip in the tofu from the skillet.

Pour in 4⅓ cups water. Bring to a boil, then reduce the heat to
a simmer. Add the bok choy and mushrooms, then immediately
remove from the heat.

Divide the udon noodles into serving bowls. Put the bok choy,
mushrooms and tofu on top of the noodles, then cover with the
miso and enoki cooking liquids. Sprinkle with the toasted sesame
seeds and add the chives, then serve.

Gluten-free Soy-free Nut-free Seed-free Sugar-free

spicy lentil & quinoa risotto

Serves: 4
Preparation: 15 minutes
Cooking: 1 hour

1 tablespoon olive oil or
   coconut oil
1 onion, finely chopped
2 garlic cloves, crushed
½-inch piece fresh ginger
   root, peeled and grated
½-inch piece fresh turmeric,
   peeled and grated or
   ½ teaspoon ground
   turmeric
1 teaspoon ground cumin
1 teaspoon garam masala
2 teaspoons crushed chilies
1 red chili, seeded and
   thinly sliced
1 cup tomatoes, chopped
11 ounces potatoes, cubed
scant 1½ cups red lentils,
   rinsed and drained
3¾ cups vegetable stock, plus
   extra if needed
½ cup red or white quinoa,
   rinsed and drained
2 ounces broccoli florets, cut
   in half
4 ounces kale, roughly
   chopped
¼ cup lemon juice
1 handful of chopped
   cilantro
dairy-free yogurt, to serve

Heat the oil in a large pot over medium-low heat. Add the onion, garlic, ginger and fresh turmeric, if using, and cook 5 to 8 minutes, stirring frequently, until softened.

Add the ground turmeric, if using, plus the cumin, garam masala, crushed chilies and fresh chili, and cook 30 seconds. Add the tomatoes, potatoes, lentils and 2⅔ cups of the stock, and bring to a gentle boil. Reduce the heat to medium-low and simmer 30 minutes, or until the liquid is absorbed.

Add ¾ cup of the stock and the quinoa, and simmer 10 minutes. Add more stock, if necessary, to avoid the quinoa becoming too dry. Add the broccoli and kale, and continue cooking 5 minutes, or until the quinoa is tender and translucent. Stir in the lemon juice and cilantro, then ladle into serving bowls and top with a large spoonful of dairy-free yogurt.

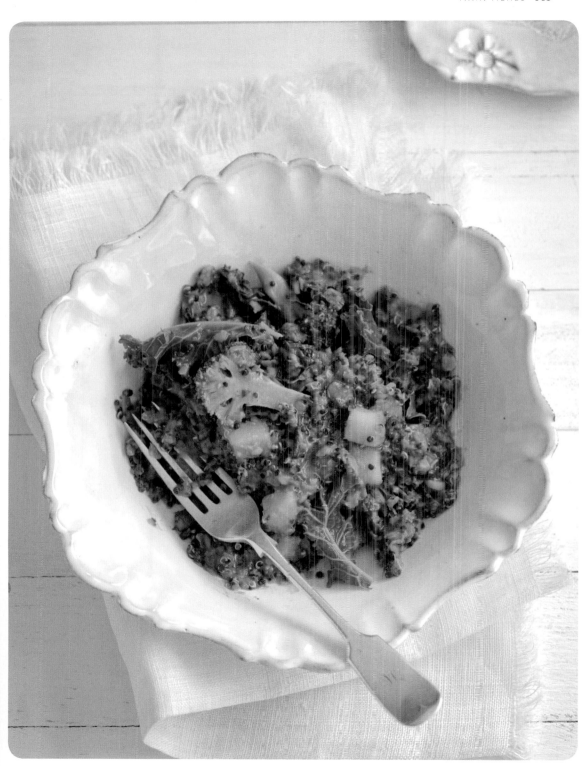

hungarian stew with garlic croutons

Serves: 4
Preparation: 30 minutes
Cooking: 45 minutes

1 tablespoon olive oil or
  coconut oil
4 large potatoes, cubed
1 large onion, chopped
1 red bell pepper, seeded
  and chopped
1 green bell pepper, seeded
  and chopped
1½ teaspoons caraway seeds
2 cups canned chopped
  tomatoes
1 cup canned lima beans,
  rinsed and drained
1 cup vegetable stock
2 teaspoons sweet paprika
½ cup walnuts, chopped
sea salt and freshly ground
  black pepper
steamed green vegetables,
  to serve

GARLIC CROUTONS
4 slices of stale sourdough
  bread
2 garlic cloves, crushed
extra virgin olive oil

Heat the oil in a large pot over medium heat. Add the potatoes and cook 8 to 10 minutes, stirring frequently, until browned all over. Add the onion, peppers and caraway seeds, and cook another 10 minutes.

Add the tomatoes, lima beans, stock and sweet paprika, then season with salt and pepper. Simmer 25 minutes, or until the potatoes are tender.

Meanwhile, to make the croutons, spread the bread with the garlic, then cut into cubes. Put in a bowl and drizzle the olive oil over them. Toss to mix, then fry in a nonstick skillet until golden, turning to brown on all sides.

Ladle the stew into bowls and top with the walnuts and croutons. Add a grinding of black pepper and serve with green vegetables.

Although this dish, called *fasolakia*, is traditionally served as an accompaniment, I have added cannellini beans to make it into a substantial meal.

greek beans with *tomatoes*

Serves: 4
Preparation: 15 minutes
Cooking: 1 hour

1 tablespoon olive oil or rice bran oil
1 onion, finely chopped
2 garlic cloves, crushed
4 cups canned chopped tomatoes
scant 6 cups canned cannellini beans, rinsed and drained
2 tablespoons chopped dill leaves
2 tablespoons thyme leaves
½ cup vegetable stock, plus extra if needed
1 pound green beans
2 tablespoons extra virgin olive oil
crusty bread or cooked quinoa, to serve

Heat the oil in a large pot over medium heat. Add the onion and garlic, and cook 5 to 8 minutes until softened.

Add the tomatoes and cannellini beans, and stir to combine. Add the dill and thyme, then pour in ½ cup stock. Stir then simmer 40 minutes, stirring occasionally. Add the green beans and cook 10 minutes, or until they are tender. Add a little more liquid if the mixture sticks to the pan. Remove from the heat and drizzle with the olive oil. Serve with crusty bread.

    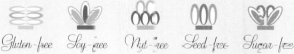

Gluten-free Soy-free Nut-free Seed-free Sugar-free

Soy-free   Sugar-free

rustic tart with *spinach pesto*

Serves: 4
Preparation: 30 minutes
Cooking: 1 hour 15 minutes

6 ounces sweet potato, thinly
  sliced into circles
1 baby beet, thinly sliced
2/3 cup peeled and cubed
  butternut squash
1 carrot, sliced
1 large onion, cut into thin
  wedges
1 tablespoon safflower oil or
  sunflower oil
6 asparagus spears
1 sheet of vegan ready-
  rolled puff pastry dough,
  defrosted if frozen
15 cherry tomatoes, cut
  in half
1/2 cup hazelnuts, chopped
green salad, to serve

TOMATO SPREAD
3 tablespoons olive oil or
  melted coconut oil
2 garlic cloves
3/4 cup drained sun-dried
  tomatoes in oil
1 teaspoon dried thyme

SPINACH PESTO
2 cups baby spinach leaves
1 handful of parsley leaves
2 tablespoons extra virgin
  olive oil
sea salt and freshly ground
  black pepper

Preheat the oven to 400°F. Put the sweet potato on a baking
sheet and add the beet, squash, carrot and onion, then drizzle
with the oil. Roast 45 minutes.

Meanwhile, snap off any woody ends from the asparagus stalks
at the point where they break easily, then cut the tender spears
into short pieces. Set to one side.

Put all the ingredients for the tomato spread into a blender or
food processor and blend until smooth. Set aside.

To make the spinach pesto, put all the ingredients in a blender or
food processor and blend until finely chopped. Add a little water
if the mixture is too thick.

After 45 minutes of roasting the vegetables, add the asparagus
to the baking sheet and roast another 10 minutes. Remove the
baking sheet from the oven and set aside.

Lay the pastry dough on a clean baking sheet, and spread with
the tomato spread, leaving a 1½-inch border. Arrange the
vegetables in a pile in the center of the pastry dough, and gently
fold in the edges to make a pastry border. Scatter the cherry
tomatoes over it. Bake the tart 15 minutes, or until the pastry
is golden brown. Drizzle the tart with the spinach pesto, then
sprinkle with the chopped nuts. Serve with a big green salad.

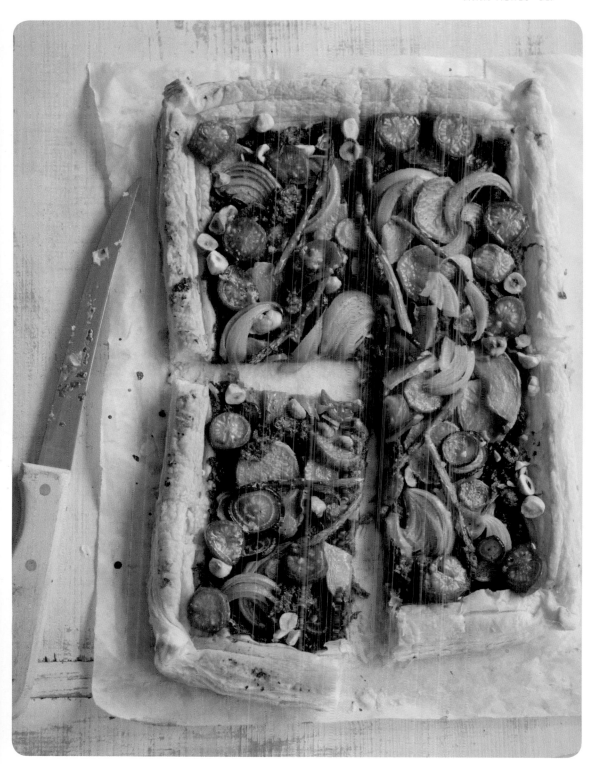

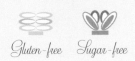

Gluten-free   Sugar-free

red lentil & beet burgers

Serves: 4
Preparation: 20 minutes, plus
**   1 hour chilling (if time),**
**   plus making the relish**
Cooking: 35 minutes

heaped ½ cup red lentils,
    rinsed and drained
1 small beet, roughly
    chopped
½ onion, roughly chopped
1 garlic clove, crushed
½ tablespoon tamari soy
    sauce, soy sauce or coconut
    aminos
1 small handful of parsley
    leaves, chopped
1 teaspoon crushed chilies
    (optional)
½ teaspoon sweet paprika
3 tablespoons coconut milk,
    plus extra if needed
¾ cup gram flour or all-
    purpose flour, plus extra if
    needed
1 tablespoon safflower oil,
    or sunflower oil, olive oil or
    coconut oil
sea salt and freshly ground
    black pepper

TO SERVE
4 wholewheat rolls
romaine lettuce leaves
sliced large tomato
Tomato Relish (page 48)
pickles

Put the lentils in a saucepan with 4⅓ cups boiling water and
return to a boil over high heat. Reduce the heat to medium
and cook 10 to 12 minutes until soft. Drain in a colander and
set aside.

Meanwhile, put the beet and onion into a food processor and
blend until finely chopped. Set to one side.

Tip the lentils into a large bowl and add the beet mixture. Stir
together to combine. Put the garlic in a small bowl and add the
tamari, parsley, crushed chilies, if using, and paprika. Season
with salt and pepper, then stir together to combine. Stir into
the lentil mixture.

Pour in 3 tablespoons coconut milk, and half the flour. Stir well
and then add the remaining flour. The consistency should be
firm enough to hold its shape without being too dry, and this will
depend on the liquid quantity from the beet. If it is too wet, add
more flour, 1 teaspoon at a time. If it is too dry, add more coconut
milk, 1 teaspoon at a time. If you have time, chill the mixture in the
refrigerator 1 hour.

Divide the mixture into 4 and form each into a burger shape.
Heat the oil in a nonstick skillet over medium-high heat.
Cook the burgers in the oil 5 to 6 minutes on each side, until
lightly golden—you may need to do this in batches. Serve with
wholewheat rolls, salad, relish and pickles.

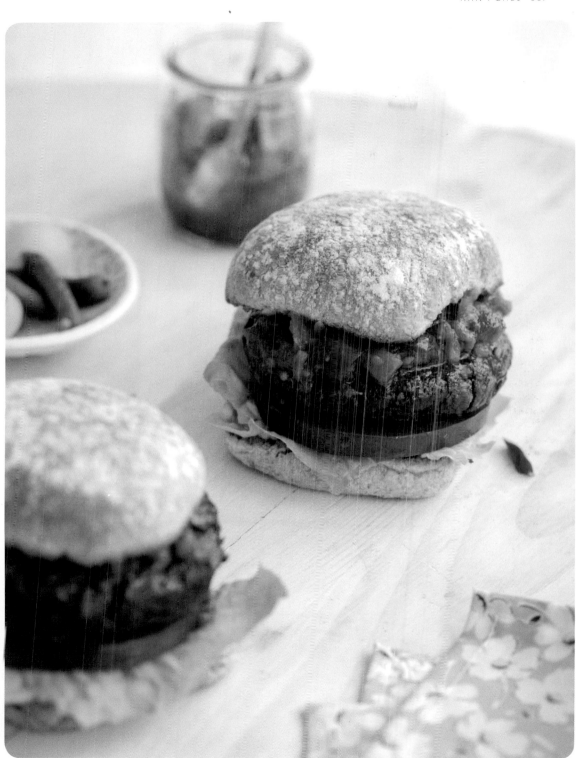

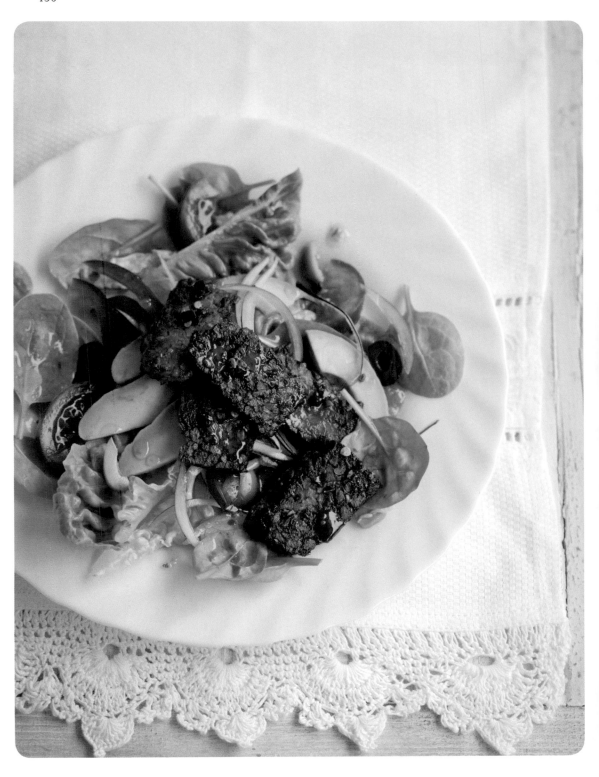

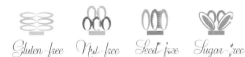

Gluten-free   *Nut-free*   *Seed-free*   *Sugar-free*

spicy warm tempeh salad

Serves 4
Preparation: 20 minutes
Cooking: 10 minutes

3 tablespoons tamari soy
 sauce or soy sauce
½ teaspoon smoked paprika
2 teaspoons crushed chilies
1 pound tempeh, cubed
1 tablespoon olive oil or
 safflower oil
2 red onions, finely sliced
1 head lettuce, leaves
 chopped
3 cups baby spinach leaves
½ red bell pepper, seeded
 and sliced
½ cup pitted green and black
 olives, sliced
2 plum or vine tomatoes, cut
 into thin wedges
2 avocados, cut in half,
 pitted, peeled and sliced

CHILI DRESSING
¼ cup olive oil
2 tablespoons lemon juice
1 tablespoon chili sauce
freshly ground black pepper

Put the tamari in a bowl and add the smoked paprika and
crushed chilies. Add the tempeh and mix well to combine, then
set aside. Heat the oil in a nonstick skillet over medium heat.
Add the tempeh and cook 5 to 8 minutes until golden brown.

Meanwhile, put the onions in a large serving bowl and add the
lettuce, spinach, pepper, olives, tomatoes and avocados. Gently
mix together, taking care not to mash the avocados.

Put all the ingredients for the dressing in a screwtop jar, cover
and shake well to combine. (Alternatively, whisk in a small bowl.)
Serve the tempeh with the salad and drizzle it with the dressing.

This dish is based on an authentic, smoky, vegan gumbo I tasted in the US. Using a slow cooker gives the gumbo a rich sauce and is my preferred method, but you can also make it in a pot on the stove cooked over very low heat.

slow - cooked smoky gumbo

Serves: 6
Preparation: 20 minutes
Cooking: 4¼ to 7¼ hours in a slow cooker or 1¾ hours in a pot on the stove

2 tablespoons olive oil or coconut oil
1 onion, chopped
3 garlic cloves, crushed
1 red bell pepper, seeded and thinly sliced
1 green bell pepper, seeded and thinly sliced
2 celery stalks, thinly sliced
4 cups canned chopped tomatoes
2 cups canned red kidney beans, rinsed and drained
1 teaspoon smoked paprika
½ teaspoon sweet paprika
½ teaspoon dried thyme
¾ cup easy-cook short grain brown rice, or jasmine or basmati rice
3 cups vegetable stock
sea salt and freshly ground black pepper
chopped cilantro and chili sauce, to serve

Heat 1 tablespoon of the oil in a nonstick skillet over medium heat and cook the onion and garlic 5 to 8 minutes until softened. Add the peppers and celery, and cook another 5 minutes, stirring frequently.

Meanwhile, if using a slow cooker, preheat it to High. Put the remaining oil in the slow cooker. Transfer the pepper mixture to the slow cooker and add the remaining ingredients. Season with salt and pepper and stir well. Cook 5 to 7 hours on Low or 4 to 6 hours on High until the rice is cooked.

If using a pot on the stove, heat the remaining oil in a large pot over medium heat, then transfer the pepper mixture to the pot. Add the remaining ingredients, season with salt and pepper, and stir well. Bring to a boil, then reduce the heat to very low and simmer very gently 1½ hours, or until the rice is cooked.

Top up with boiling water if the mixture becomes too dry. The gumbo should look like a thick soup. Scatter the cilantro over it and serve with the chili sauce.

Gluten-free *Soy-free* *Nut-free* *Seed-free* *Sugar-free*

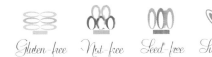

Gluten-free   Nut-free   Seed-free   Sugar-free

vegetable slice with chimichurri
& tomato salsa

Serves 4
**Preparation: 20 minutes,
  plus 1 hour resting**
Cooking: 1 hour

1 tablespoon olive oil or
  safflower oil, plus extra for
  greasing
1 onion, chopped
4 garlic cloves, crushed
2 zucchini, coarsely grated
4 cups baby spinach
11 ounces firm tofu
⅓ cup soy milk
2 teaspoons cornstarch or
  arrowroot
6 ounces broccoli, chopped
½ red bell pepper, seeded
  and chopped
sea salt and freshly ground
  black pepper

TOMATO SALSA
2 large ripe tomatoes,
  chopped
½ onion, chopped
juice of 2 limes
1 large handful of cilantro,
  chopped

CHIMICHURRI
¼ cup parsley leaves
1 garlic clove
½ teaspoon dried oregano
2 tablespoons olive oil
1 teaspoon vinegar
¼ teaspoon crushed chilies

To make the salsa, put all the ingredients in a serving bowl and add a pinch of salt. Mix well and set aside 1 hour for the flavors to develop.

Preheat the oven to 350°F and grease a 9 x 9-inch nonstick baking pan with a little oil. Heat the oil in a nonstick pot over medium heat. Add the onion and garlic, and cook 5 to 8 minutes until softened. Add the zucchini to the pot, stir well and cook 5 minutes, stirring occasionally.

Put the spinach in a blender or food processor and add the tofu, soy milk and cornstarch, then blend until smooth. Add the zucchini and onion mixture, the broccoli and red bell pepper. Season with salt and pepper then pulse quickly to combine roughly, leaving some noticeable pieces of pepper and broccoli.

Pour the mixture into the prepared baking pan and bake 45 minutes, or until firm and golden. Meanwhile, to make the chimichurri, put the parsley in a food processor and add the remaining ingredients. Blend until they form a paste. Spoon into a serving bowl and set aside. Serve the vegetable slice with the chimichurri and salsa

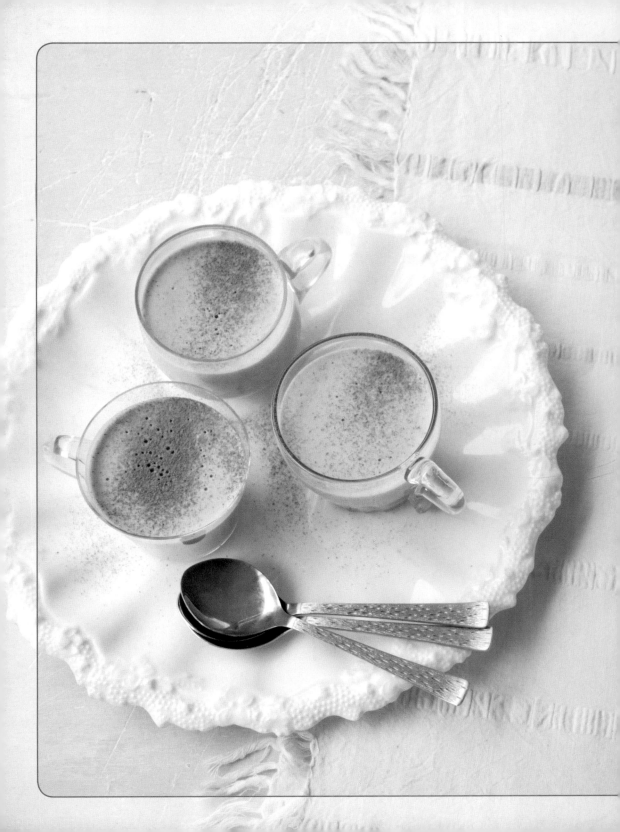

Desserts

The part of the meal I look forward to the most—desserts!
I love making them too, not just for the burst of sweetness
but for the chance to experiment with new flavors and
techniques. Here, I have made traditional desserts with a
fresh twist, and healthier versions of time-honored favorites.
Brighten your palate with a fruit granita or sherbet, such
as Strawberry & Hibiscus Flower Granita, or finish your
meal with the creamy texture of Coconut Kulfi Ice Cream
or Rosewater & Pistachio Syllabub. Transform a fresh fruit
salad with a touch of Thai by making Fruit Salad with
Strawberry & Lemongrass Syrup or liven up pineapple by
making Grilled Chili Pineapple with Mint & Yogurt. And for
a twist on a traditional cheesecake, try my Raw Chocolate
Torte with Salted Pecan Sauce.

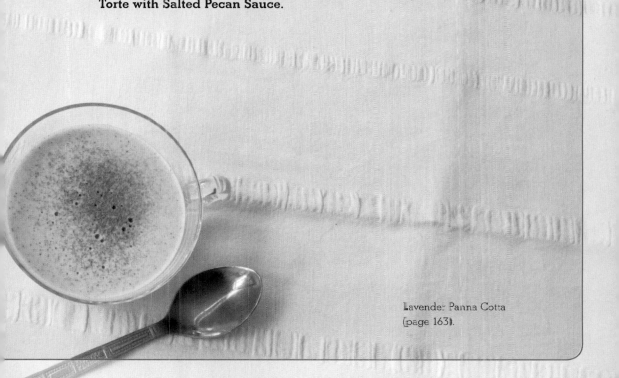

Lavender Panna Cotta
(page 163).

Hibiscus flower tea is drunk as a traditional herbal remedy in several countries—in Egypt to support a healthy heart and nervous system, in Mexico as a diuretic, in Asia to help lower cholesterol and in the Middle East to relieve restlessness. It has a beautiful scent and flavor, and it complements the flavor of strawberries perfectly in this sweet granita.

strawberry & *hibiscus flower granita*

Serves: 6
Preparation: 5 minutes,
   plus 15 minutes infusing,
   cooling, 10 minutes chilling
   and 2½ hours freezing

2 tablespoons dried hibiscus
   flower tea
1 pound, 5 ounces
   strawberries, hulled, plus
   extra strawberries, cut in
   half, for decorating
2 tablespoons lime juice
1 tablespoon brown rice
   syrup or agave syrup
1 teaspoon syrup from a jar of
   hibiscus flowers (optional)

Put the hibiscus flower tea in a bowl and add 1½ cups boiling water. Let infuse 15 minutes, then let cool and chill in the refrigerator 10 minutes.

Put the tea into a blender or food processor and add the strawberries, lime juice and brown rice syrup. Blend well. Add the hibiscus syrup, if using, then blend briefly to mix.

Pour into a shallow freezerproof container. Put in the freezer 30 minutes, then scrape the mixture with a fork to break up the ice crystals slightly.

Repeat the freezing and scraping another 4 times, or until the granita is frozen throughout with fine, even crystals. Serve in glasses and top with halved strawberries.

Gluten-free   Soy-free   Nut-free   Seed-free   Raw

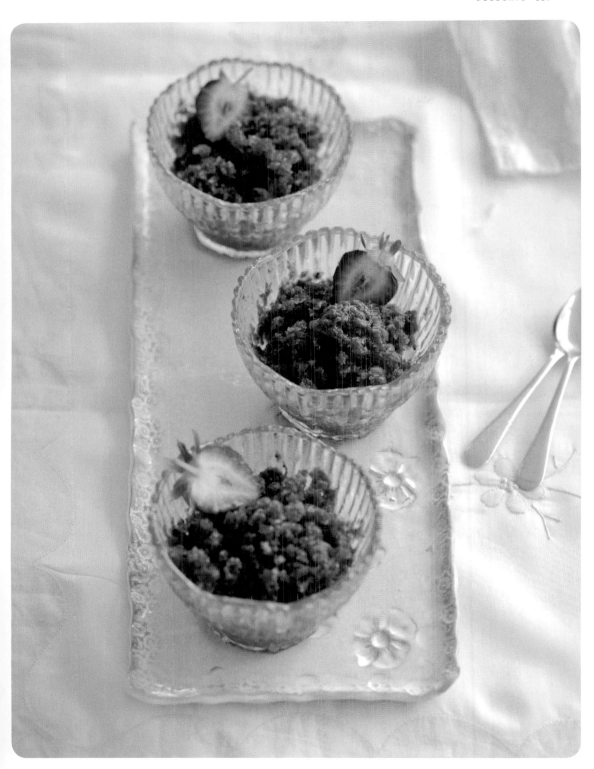

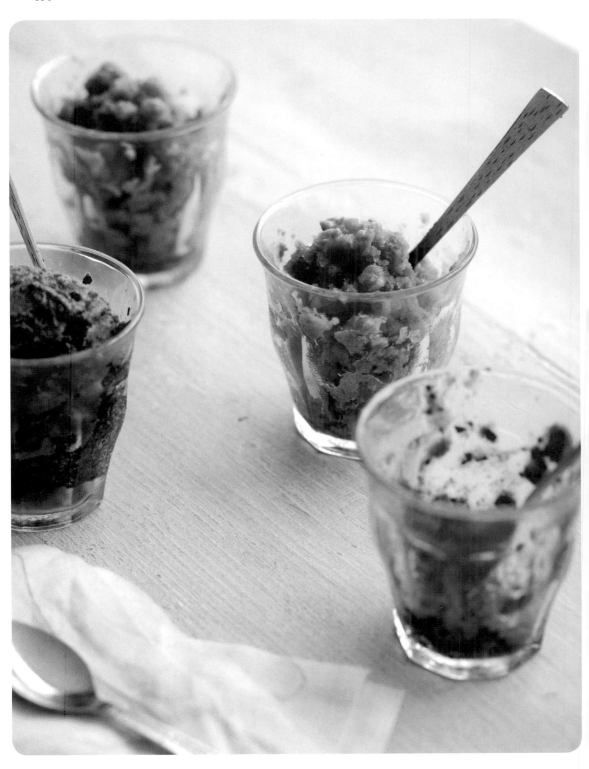

lychee, raspberry & *rose sherbet*

Serves: 6
Preparation: 15 minutes,
  plus 4 hours freezing and
  20 minutes defrosting

3⅓ cups canned lychees
  in syrup
1 cup raspberries
1 teaspoon rose water
basil leaves, to serve
  (optional)

Put the lychees and their syrup into a blender or food processor and add the remaining ingredients. Blend until smooth. Pour into a shallow freezerproof container and put into the freezer 2 hours, or until the mixture is frozen around the edges.

Using an electric beater, a blender or food processor, beat to break up the crystals, then refreeze another 1 hour, or until crystals form. Beat again and freeze until solid. Defrost at room temperature 20 minutes before serving, with basil, if you like.

Gluten-free *Soy-free* *Nut-free* *Seed-free*

plum, black pepper & *vanilla sherbet*

Serves: 4
Preparation: 15 minutes, plus
  overnight and an additional
  4 hours freezing and
  20 minutes defrosting

6 ripe sweet, dark plums,
  pitted and cut into quarters
½ vanilla bean
½ teaspoon black
  peppercorns

Put the plums in a freezer bag, seal and freeze overnight.

Split the vanilla bean in half lengthwise and scrape out the seeds. Reserve the bean for another use. Put the vanilla seeds, plums and peppercorns into a blender or food processor and blend until smooth and creamy. Serve immediately, or freeze 3 to 4 hours to harden. Defrost at room temperature 20 minutes and blend briefly before serving.

Gluten-free *Soy-free* *Nut-free* *Seed-free* *Sugar-free* *Raw*

coconut kulfi ice cream (pictured)

Serves 4
Preparation: 15 minutes,
plus 4 hours freezing

3½ cups coconut cream
¼ cup coconut oil, melted
1 cup brown sugar or
coconut sugar
½ cup pistachios, plus extra
chopped pistachios to serve
1 teaspoon ground
cardamom

Put all the ingredients into a blender or food processor and blend until smooth. Pour into a shallow freezerproof container and freeze 3 to 4 hours or until almost solid.

Return to the blender and blend until smooth. (Alternatively, pour into an ice cream maker and follow the manufacturer's instructions.) Serve topped with nuts.

Gluten-free *Soy-free* *Seed-free*

raw maple pecan ice cream

Serves 4
Preparation: 10 minutes,
plus overnight freezing

4 ripe bananas, chopped
1 vanilla bean
⅓ cup raw almond butter
½ cup raw tahini
¾ cup maple syrup or ¾ cup
brown sugar or coconut
sugar
1 teaspoon ground cinnamon
1½ cups pecans, chopped

Unless you have an ice cream maker, put the banana pieces in a freezer bag, seal and freeze overnight.

Split the vanilla bean in half lengthwise and scrape out the seeds. Reserve the bean for another use. Put all the ingredients into a high-speed blender or food processor and blend until smooth. (Alternatively, blend all the ingredients in a blender or food processor until smooth, then transfer to an ice cream maker and follow the manufacturer's instructions.) Serve immediately.

Gluten-free *Soy-free* *Raw*

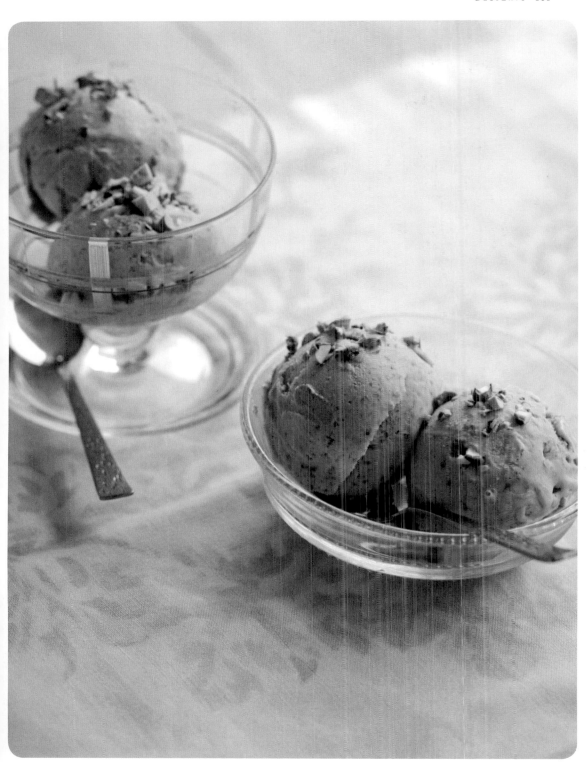

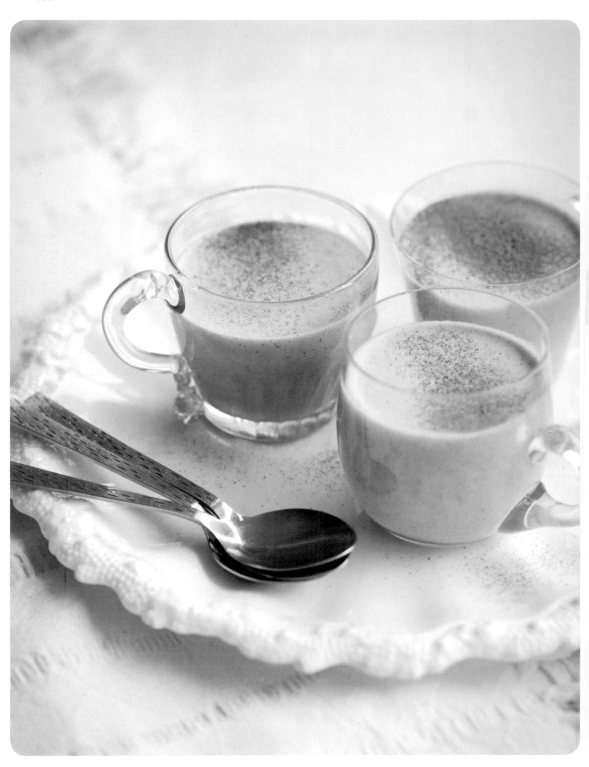

A traditional Italian dessert, panna cotta is normally made with milk, cream and gelatin. My version, with its delicate floral flavor, is a delicious, light and creamy dessert that you wouldn't believe is vegan. If you have never cooked with agar—the vegetarian alternative to gelatin—before, it's very easy to use and has no taste or color.

lavender panna cotta

Serves: 4
Preparation: 10 minutes
Cooking: 15 minutes, plus
  cooling and overnight
  chilling

1 vanilla bean
2 teaspoons culinary lavender
  flowers
2 cups coconut milk
2 tablespoons brown sugar or
  coconut sugar
½ teaspoon ground
  cinnamon, plus extra for
  sprinkling
2 teaspoons agar flakes

Split the vanilla bean in half lengthwise and scrape out the seeds. Reserve the bean for another use. Using the back of a spoon, crush the lavender flowers.

Put the coconut milk in a small saucepan over low heat and add the vanilla seeds, lavender, sugar and cinnamon. Bring gently to a boil, then simmer. Add the agar and 2 tablespoons water, and continue to simmer until the agar has dissolved completely and no trace of the flakes can be seen when you lift up some of the mixture in a spoon.

Divide the mixture into four individual ramekins or small glasses. Let cool, then put into the refrigerator to set overnight. Serve sprinkled with cinnamon.

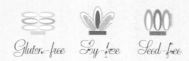

Gluten-free Soy-free Seed-free

A syllabub is an old-fashioned English dessert that is traditionally made with cream and wine. It's like a beautifully creamy mousse. My vegan version is just as rich, but it's healthier and made with coconut cream, pistachios and cashews with the delicate flavor of rosewater.

rosewater & *pistachio syllabub*

Serves: 4
Preparation: 15 minutes,
  plus overnight chilling
  and soaking

1 cup coconut cream in the
  unopened carton or can
scant 2 cups cashews
½ cup pistachios, plus
  chopped pistachios to serve
1 tablespoon brown sugar or
  coconut sugar
1 to 2 teaspoons rosewater
rose petals, to serve

Chill the coconut cream overnight in the refrigerator, making sure the carton is upright. Put the cashews in a bowl, cover with water and let soak overnight. Drain in a colander, then rinse well and drain again.

Put the pistachios into a food processor and grind until fine but without becoming oily. Set aside.

Without shaking the carton of coconut cream, open it and scoop off ½ cup of the cream from the top—it will be very, very thick. Put ¼ cup of the liquid from the carton in a small bowl. Store the remaining cream and liquid in a covered container in the refrigerator for another use.

Put the coconut cream into a blender or food processor and add the cashews, sugar and rosewater, to taste. Blend until smooth. Add the reserved liquid, 1 tablespoon at a time, if needed, to make the cream soft but thick enough to hold its shape. Pour into a bowl and add the ground pistachios. Spoon into four glasses, and serve sprinkled with chopped pistachios and rose petals.

Gluten-free　　*Soy-free*　　*Seed-free*

Gluten-free Soy-free Seed-free

fruit salad with strawberry & lemongrass syrup

Serves: 4
Preparation: 20 minutes
**Cooking: 5 minutes, plus
5 minutes cooling**

1 cup brown sugar or
coconut sugar
2 lemongrass stalks, outer
leaves removed, bruised
with a knife
1 cup strawberries, hulled
2 teaspoons lime juice
1 banana, sliced
2 kiwifruits, peeled and
cubed
6 ounces watermelon,
cubed
6 ounces cantaloupe, cubed
1 cup seedless green grapes
1 cup coconut cream

Put 1½ cups water in a small saucepan over medium heat and add the sugar, lemongrass and strawberries. Bring gently to a boil, then reduce the heat to low and simmer 4 to 5 minutes, stirring occasionally, until the sugar is dissolved.

Remove the lemongrass and mash the strawberries using a fork. Whisk in the lime juice then let cool 5 minutes.

Put the banana slices in a serving bowl and add the kiwifruit, watermelon, cantaloupe and grapes. Add the strawberry and lemongrass syrup, and stir gently to combine. Serve drizzled with coconut cream.

Serve these spiced pears with creamy coconut yogurt or slice them and serve for breakfast to top the Toasted Granola on page 36. You can also slice or cube the pears before cooking, if you prefer.

chai-poached pears

Serves: 6
Preparation: 10 minutes
Cooking: 1 hour

¾ cup brown sugar or
  coconut sugar
1 tablespoon lemon juice
1 teaspoon cardamom
  pods, crushed
3 cloves
2 cinnamon sticks
1 star anise
½ teaspoon grated nutmeg
a pinch of sea salt
3 medium pears, peeled,
  stalks intact
dairy-free yogurt, to serve

Put the sugar in a medium saucepan and add 1 cup water, the lemon juice, spices and salt. Bring to just boiling over medium heat and then reduce the heat to a simmer. Stir well to dissolve the sugar. Turn the heat to low, and add the pears, stirring well to ensure the syrup covers them. Top up with water to cover if necessary. Cook 30 minutes, or until the pears are tender—the cooking time will depend on the ripeness of the pears.

Remove the pears with a slotted spoon. If you like, you can reduce the remainder of the chai syrup by increasing the heat after the pears have been removed, and cooking another 15 to 25 minutes until thick. Serve the pears with yogurt, and with the reduced juice drizzled over the top, if you like.

Gluten-free

Soy-free

Nut-free

Seed-free

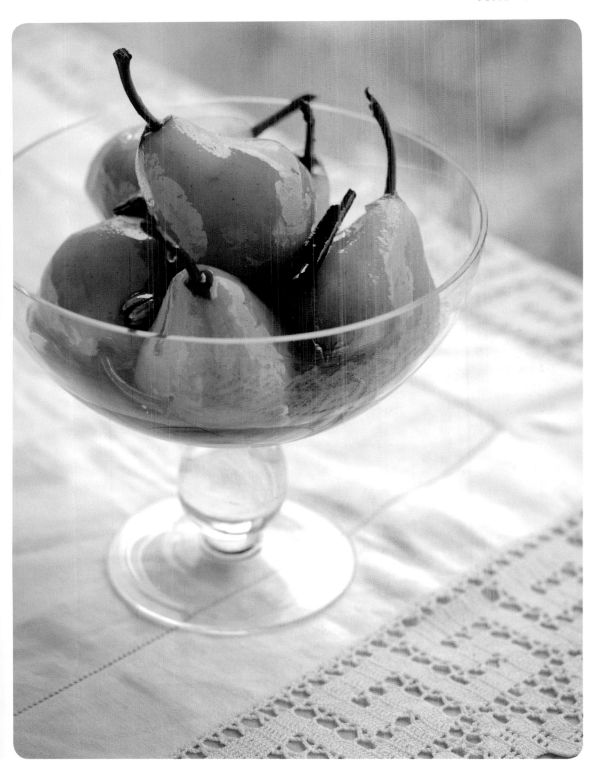

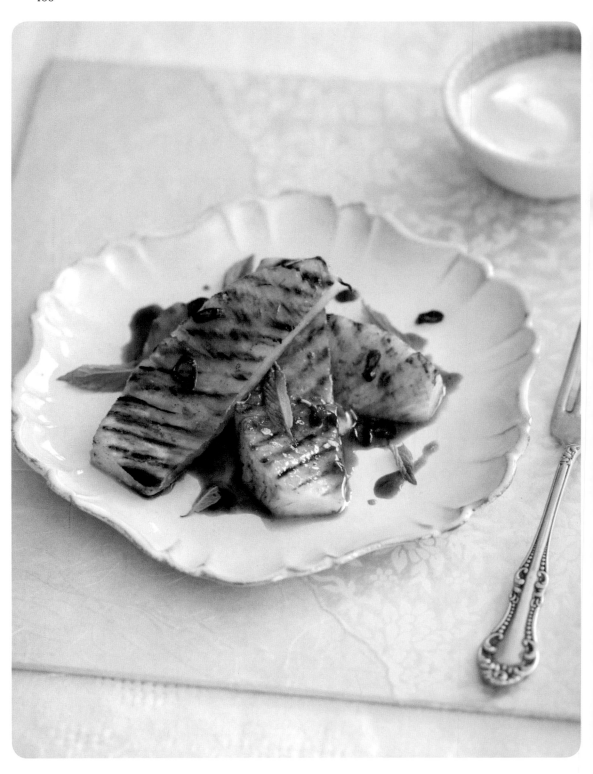

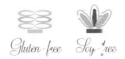

Gluten-free *Soy-free*

grilled chili pineapple
with mint & yogurt

Serves: 4
Preparation: 15 minutes
Cooking: 15 minutes

1 large pineapple
2 tablespoons brown sugar or
   coconut sugar
½ hot red chili, such as Thai
   chili, seeded and finely
   chopped
1 teaspoon ground cinnamon
1 tablespoon safflower oil,
   sunflower oil or coconut oil
a few small mint leaves
1 cup dairy-free coconut
   yogurt

Cut the top and bottom off the pineapple and stand it up on a cutting board. Slice off the skin, cutting downwards from top to bottom. Carefully cut out any pieces of skin left on the fruit. Cut the pineapple in half lengthwise and then in half again, then slice off the woody core so that you are left with the soft fruit. Slice each quarter in half lengthwise.

Put the sugar, chili and cinnamon in a small saucepan over medium-low heat, and heat through to dissolve the sugar.

Heat a large, ridged grill pan over medium-high heat. Brush both sides of the pineapple with the oil and cook the pineapple in the grill pan 5 to 6 minutes, turning once, until it is warmed through and is marked with golden lines. You may have to do this in batches. Remove from the grill pan and keep warm.

Meanwhile, increase the heat under the saucepan to medium-high to lightly caramelize the sugar. Transfer the pineapple to serving plates, pour the sauce over the top and scatter the mint leaves over it. Serve with the yogurt.

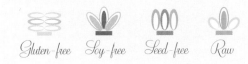

Gluten-free *Soy-free* *Seed-free* *Raw*

raw chocolate torte with
salted pecan sauce

Serves: 8
Preparation: 30 minutes
  plus overnight soaking,
  4 to 5 hours freezing and
  20 minutes defrosting

2¼ cups cashews
1 vanilla bean
⅔ cup coconut sugar
scant 1 cup raw cacao
  powder
½ teaspoon sea salt
scant ¾ cup coconut oil,
  melted
raw chocolate shavings and
  mixed berries, to serve

SALTED PECAN SAUCE
1 cup fresh or dried medjool
  dates, pitted
1 cup pecans
¼ cup agave syrup or brown
  rice syrup
1 teaspoon sea salt

DATE CRUST
½ cup fresh or dried medjool
  dates, pitted
1½ cups almonds
a pinch of sea salt

Put the cashews in a bowl, cover with water and let soak overnight. Drain in a colander and rinse. Meanwhile, put the dates and pecans for the sauce in a bowl. Put the dried dates, if using, for the crust into another bowl. Cover both with water, and let soak 4 hours. Drain and rinse the nuts. Drain the dates for the crust, but drain and reserve the date liquid for the sauce.

To make the crust, put the almonds, dates and salt into a blender or food processor and blend at high speed to form a soft dough. Press the dough lightly into the bottom of an 8-inch springform pan and let chill in the refrigerator while you make the filling.

Split the vanilla bean in half lengthwise and scrape out the seeds. Reserve the bean for another use. Put the vanilla seeds, sugar, cacao powder, salt and oil into a blender or food processor and add ¾ cup water. Blend until smooth. Pour this filling over the crust. Freeze the cake 4 to 5 hours until firm.

To make the sauce, put all the ingredients into a blender or food processor and blend until smooth, adding the reserved date liquid, 1 tablespoon at a time, until the sauce is thick and creamy. Remove the torte from the freezer, then carefully release the sides of the pan and slide the torte onto a serving plate. Leave 20 minutes to defrost slightly. Drizzle the sauce over the top and scatter the chocolate shavings and mixed berries over it, then serve.

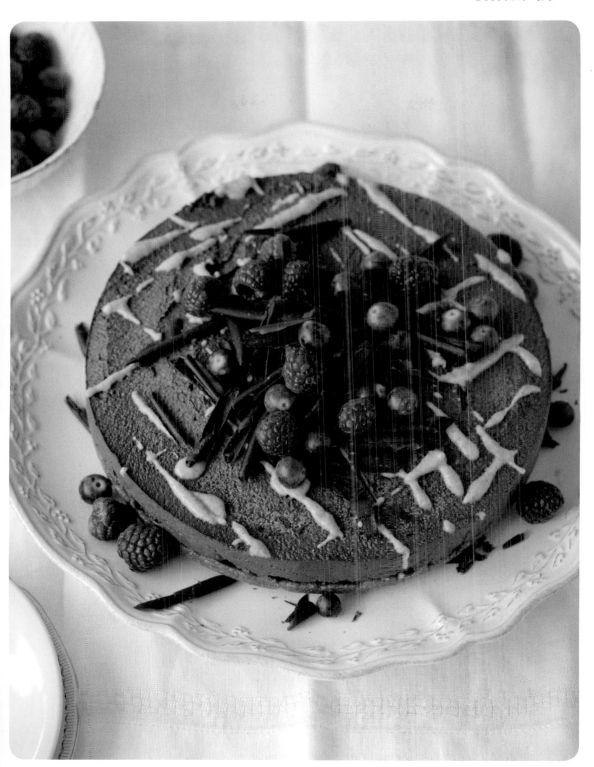

A fast and easy dessert made with little mouthfuls of chocolate melted through banana in a rice wrapper.

chocolate banana wontons

Serves: 6
Preparation: 25 minutes
Cooking: 20 minutes

1 pack of 30 egg-free vegan wonton wrappers
2 large ripe bananas, chopped
3 ounces dark vegan chocolate, chopped, plus extra chocolate, grated, to serve
¼ cup safflower oil, sunflower oil or coconut oil, plus extra if needed

Preheat the oven to 200°F and put a large heatproof plate inside to warm. Separate the wonton wrappers and lay them on a damp dish towel. This will prevent them from drying out.

Put the bananas in a large bowl and add the dark chocolate, then mix together well. Spoon a small teaspoonful of the banana mixture onto each wonton wrapper. Moisten the edges with a little water and fold into a triangle. Leave them on the damp dish towel and continue until all the wonton wrappers are used.

Heat 2 tablespoons of the oil in a large, nonstick skillet and cook 2 or 3 wontons at a time, allowing them to turn golden brown and bubble a little on the surface. Remove with a slotted spoon and drain on paper towels. Keep the wontons warm while you cook the rest, adding oil as necessary. Serve sprinkled with grated chocolate.

Nut-free

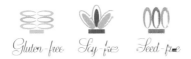

Gluten-free Soy-free Seed-free

banana-leaf mango *rice cakes*

Serves: 4
Preparation: 20 minutes
Cooking: 40 minutes, plus
20 minutes cooling

1 cup glutinous (sticky) rice
1 cup coconut milk, plus
  extra to serve
½ teaspoon sea salt
¼ cup brown sugar or
  coconut sugar
2 bananas, chopped
1 small mango, peeled and
  pitted, flesh chopped (about
  2¾ ounces flesh)
1 pound banana leaves,
  defrosted if frozen (8 leaves)
  (or use foil, if unavailable)
black sesame seeds, to serve

Put the rice in a saucepan over medium-high heat and add the coconut milk, 1 cup water, the salt and sugar. Stir together, then bring to a boil. Reduce the heat to low and cook 20 minutes, stirring frequently, or until the rice is plump and the liquid is absorbed. Remove from the heat and let cool 20 minutes.

Preheat the oven to 400°F and line a baking tray with baking parchment. When the rice is cool enough to handle, add the bananas and mango to the pan and gently stir to combine.

Lay a banana leaf out flat and take a large tablespoonful of the rice mixture. Form it into a ball and put it on the banana leaf near to the top edge. Roll up the banana leaf, tucking in the sides neatly. Tie some kitchen string around the banana roll to hold it securely, then put the roll on the prepared baking tray. (Alternatively, grease a small rectangle of foil with a little oil and wrap the rice up as before, sealing the edges well.) Repeat with the remaining rice and banana leaves.

Cook in the oven 15 to 20 minutes until the banana leaf starts to turn black. Remove each wrap with tongs and put on a serving plate, then cut off the string. Serve the rice cakes in the banana leaves (but take the rice out of the foil for serving). Be careful of the steam when opening the wraps. Sprinkle each rice cake with sesame seeds. Enjoy right from the oven with extra coconut milk drizzled over the top, or serve cooled.

index

Acknowledgments

I would like to thank my dear husband Paul for eating my creations, and even though your two least favorite dishes are soup and curry, you still eat them with love and appreciation—thank you my love. I would also like to thank my parents, Shirley and Steven, for instilling a love of good food in me from a young age, and for being amazing home cooks. Thanks to Charlie and Hank, my fur-babies, for eating everything with gusto (even the failed attempts), and to Grace, Manisha and my editor, Jan, at Duncan Baird Publishers, for holding my hand through this entire process—thank you infinitely. But most of all, thank you to all the Vegie Heads, my followers, fans, sounding boards and friends. Thank you for being you. This book proves that loving what you do, and doing what you love, can change the world.